Teaching Perinatal Care

A Practical Guide

ANNE BIRINGER, MD

SABRINA KOLKER, MD

WARREN RUBENSTEIN, MD

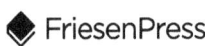 FriesenPress

One Printers Way
Altona, MB R0G 0B0
Canada

www.friesenpress.com

ISBN
978-1-03-914564-1 (Hardcover)
978-1-03-914563-4 (Paperback)
978-1-03-914565-8 (eBook)

1. Medical, Education & Training

Distributed to the trade by The Ingram Book Company

EDITORS

Anne Biringer, MD, is an associate professor in the Department of Family and Community Medicine at the University of Toronto and holds the Ada Slaight and Slaight Family Foundation Directorship in Family Medicine Maternity Care at Mount Sinai Hospital, Toronto. She practices and teaches comprehensive family medicine, including perinatal care. Her research interests include many aspects of maternity care: mental and psychosocial health, screening, clinical practice guidelines, and family medicine maternity care training. She has held many leadership positions in maternity care both locally and nationally, and regularly teaches both family medicine and obstetrics in under-resourced settings.

Sabrina Kolker, MD, is a family physician practising comprehensive family medicine, including perinatal care. She is an assistant professor in the Department of Family and Community Medicine at the University of Toronto. She is the perinatal care education lead at Toronto's Mount Sinai Hospital Academic Family Health team, where she teaches residents and medical students.

Warren Rubenstein, MD, is a family physician trained in medical education at the Family Medicine Program, Royal College of General Practitioners of Australia. He is an associate professor in the Department of Family and Community Medicine at the University of Toronto. Since 1978, he has taught medical students and residents in the teaching centre at Mount Sinai Hospital in Toronto. He is the senior author of *Medical Teaching in Ambulatory Care*, first published in 1993 and now in its third edition. In addition to English, the book has been published in French, Spanish, and Portuguese. He has presented lectures and workshops on topics focusing on teaching in ambulatory care and competency-based medical education at conferences and universities worldwide.

DEDICATIONS

To my parents and my daughters, Claire and Sarah—my teachers and my inspiration.

—A. B.

To Larry, Liam, Logan, Magalie, my mom Suzan, and my dad Bill.

And for all the teachers and coaches who have guided me.

—S. K.

To Susan and Jonathan—amor vincit omnia.

—W. R.

CONTENTS

ACKNOWLEDGEMENTS

The National Forum on Teaching Competence in Family Medicine Maternity Care and the writing of this book were supported by an unconditional donation to the Mount Sinai Academic Health Team by Ada Slaight and the Slaight Family Foundation. We are deeply grateful for their generosity.

AUTHOR LIST

Erin Bearss, MD, CCFP (EM)
Assistant Professor
Department of Family and Community Medicine, University of Toronto

Anne Biringer, MD, FCFP
Associate Professor
Department of Family and Community Medicine, University of Toronto

Tali Bogler, MD, CCFP, MScCH
Assistant Professor
Department of Family and Community Medicine, University of Toronto

David W. Eisen, MD, FCFP
Associate Professor
Department of Family and Community Medicine, University of Toronto

Perle Feldman, MDCM, FCFP, MHPE
Associate Professor
Department of Family Medicine, McGill University

Milena Forte, MD, FCFP
Associate Professor
Department of Family and Community Medicine, University of Toronto

Sabrina Kolker, MD, MSc, MA, CCFP
Assistant Professor
Department of Family and Community Medicine, University of Toronto

Natalie Morson, MD, MScCH, CCFP
Assistant Professor
Department of Family and Community Medicine, University of Toronto

Amanda Pendergast, MD, MClSci, FCFP
Associate Professor
Discipline of Family Medicine, Memorial University of Newfoundland

Warren Rubenstein, MD, FCFP
Associate Professor
Department of Family and Community Medicine, University of Toronto

Hannah Shenker, MD, CCFP
Assistant Professor
Department of Family Medicine, McGill University

Mira Shuman, MD, MScCH, CCFP
Lecturer
Department of Family and Community Medicine, University of Toronto

Kate (Katherine) Stead, MD, CCFP
Lecturer
Department of Family and Community Medicine, University of Toronto

David Tannenbaum, MD, FCFP
Associate Professor
Department of Family and Community Medicine, University of Toronto

Evan Tannenbaum, MD, MSc, FRCSC
Assistant Professor
Department of Obstetrics and Gynecology, University of Toronto

Vicki Van Wagner, RM, PhD
Associate Professor
Midwifery Education Program, Toronto Metropolitan University

Gary S. Viner, MD, MEd, FCFP
Associate Professor
Department of Family Medicine, University of Ottawa

David White, MD, FCFP
Professor
Department of Family and Community Medicine, University of Toronto

Rory Windrim, MD, MSc, FRCSC
Professor
Department of Obstetrics and Gynecology, University of Toronto

Introduction

This book is for teachers of perinatal care. The authors include family physicians, obstetricians, and a midwife, each at different stages of their clinical and educational careers. We intend for this book to be useful to all perinatal care providers and all levels of learners from different disciplines. We hope that readers see themselves in these pages, and their learners in the examples.

Why Was This Book Written?

This book originated in presentations and workshops at the National Forum on Teaching Competence in Family Medicine Maternity Care. This biennial conference held in Toronto, Canada, was started in 2014 to address the problem of dwindling participation in intrapartum care by family physicians and those learning with them. This ongoing forum provides a safe and collegial space for like-minded care providers and teachers from across Canada. The editors realized there was a tremendous amount of expertise being shared at the conference that could have wider reach in book format. Though the genesis of this book was about support for teaching family medicine perinatal care, we realized these concepts could be broadly applied in all disciplines involved in this field.

To our knowledge, there is no comprehensive text that addresses the unique features of teaching perinatal care in the office and labour and birth environment. This book focuses on the individual teacher. It is particularly suited for the clinician who may be early in their teaching career. However, we anticipate that all perinatal care teachers will find insight herein.

This book is focused on teaching techniques, not the *content* of clinical care. During the editing process, we have had to continuously remind ourselves and the chapter authors to focus on techniques. However, we have included examples in each chapter of clinical scenarios that illustrate educational principles and practice.

This is a multi-author book. The reader will notice that the chapters reflect the personalities, writing styles, and experiences of the different authors. We editors are also at different stages of our careers and have had the opportunity to reflect on how the process of reading and editing the various chapters has affected us. It has certainly made us more mindful of our own clinical teaching and appreciative of the dedication, academic rigour, and creativity of our chapter authors. As this book evolved, so did we.

The concept for the book was born prior to the COVID–19 pandemic. However, all the work was done during the pandemic—over countless Zoom meetings and individual writing sessions. Despite the added burden of being clinicians during a pandemic, the chapter authors took time to reflect on their experience and expertise and find the words to express their ideas in accessible ways. The explosion of virtual clinical care at this time also necessitated a chapter on teaching virtual perinatal care.

A Guide to This Book

Here is a brief description of what teachers might learn from each chapter. Note that each chapter opens with a teacher seeking further information about a particular area of teaching perinatal care.

1. **Teaching Perinatal Care in the Office**

   As most teaching about prenatal care occurs in the ambulatory setting, this chapter introduces the different ways in which a clinician can prepare for the participation of learners in their office. It includes guidance on the preparation of patients and office staff, including different booking strategies, as well as tips for the clinical supervision of learners.

2. **Virtual Perinatal Care: Implications for Teaching**

   Prenatal care was changed drastically when the COVID–19 pandemic arrived. In an effort to shelter pregnant people from unnecessary risk, much of prenatal care became virtual, requiring a swift pivot in clinical care. This chapter describes the implications of virtual prenatal care and tips for supervising learners in this environment.

3. **Teaching Learners About Labour and Birth**

   This chapter describes different strategies for in-the-moment teaching in labour and delivery settings. In addition to providing multiple clinical teaching opportunities, intrapartum care gives learners a chance to see their role models in action. This chapter focuses on teaching tips for procedures that often happen "in the dark," as well as other strategies for teaching learners in the high-intensity environment of the labour and delivery room.

4. **Simulation for Teaching Perinatal Care**

   Simulation has become an essential tool health professions education. This chapter describes the multiple benefits of simulation in teaching perinatal care. It focuses primarily on simple simulations, with many examples and photos. It also describes the role of high-fidelity simulation and team assessment using roleplay.

5. **Teaching Learners About Breastfeeding**

   This chapter describes multiple practical strategies to teach learners about breastfeeding at each stage of perinatal care. In addition to a review of different teaching techniques, a robust list of educational resources is provided.

6. **The Generational Divide: Impact on Teaching**

   Most perinatal care teachers are either Baby Boomers or "Gen X," whereas most learners are Millennials or "Gen Z." This chapter will help the reader understand the typical characteristics of generational cohorts, appreciate common potential tension points within them, and outline strategies to enhance teaching and learning in the perinatal care environment.

7. **Mentorship in Perinatal Care**

   Mentorship has been recognized as key to successful development in virtually every human endeavour. In this chapter, we examine different types of mentorship and the qualities and behaviours required to be a good mentor.

8. **Teaching Perinatal Care to the Uninterested Learner**

   Perinatal care is a core aspect of medical education. However, there will always be medical learners who are reluctant or uninterested because they do not anticipate incorporating perinatal care into their future practices. The educational principles in this chapter address teaching the learner uninterested in perinatal care; however, these principles can be applied to teaching in any discipline. We examine topics such as motivational theory and role-modelling.

9. **Competency-Based Education**

   Health professions are moving toward competency-based education (CBE), an educational approach that focuses on the outcomes of training. This chapter describes the principles of CBE and the use of entrustable professional activities (EPAs) in perinatal education.

10. **Evaluation**

    All teacher-learner interactions should contain an evaluative component. In this final chapter, we look at the principles of feedback and evaluation in the context of perinatal care education.

Finally, we would like to address the use of pronouns and the word "woman" in this book. We acknowledge that not all birthing people identify as women, and we have tried to standardize our language to make it inclusive. We are using the term perinatal care instead of maternity care or obstetrical care, as we consider it more inclusive of all patients and teachers.

We hope that you find this book a helpful resource in your teaching of perinatal care. The three of us have learned so much during the writing and editing process.

Anne Biringer
Sabrina Kolker
Warren Rubenstein

Chapter 1

TEACHING PERINATAL CARE IN THE OFFICE

Mira Shuman

Dr. Imelda Flores has a busy prenatal clinic and is preparing to have learners join her for the first time. She is trying to determine how to best accommodate learners, as she fears patient care may be compromised if she does not think through all the steps carefully. She is excited to integrate learners into her clinic but wants to ensure her patients continue to receive high-quality care. She opens her book on teaching in ambulatory care and finds several suggestions and teaching tips that are helpful to set up her office to welcome learners.

The majority of prenatal care occurs in an ambulatory or office setting. Given the high number of visits in any pregnancy, there are numerous opportunities for interaction and connection with learners. During this period, teachers and learners have an opportunity to participate in a unique experience as they help guide the patients through a life-changing event. They help the pregnant patient navigate important decisions throughout the pregnancy as the family prepares for their transition into parenthood.

Medical learners have acquired most of their skills and examination techniques in an inpatient hospital setting. In the inpatient setting, knowledge acquisition occurs by following a small number of patients intensively. In the ambulatory setting, this learning occurs by following a greater number of patients (Fields, 2000). Learners will develop new skill sets when participating in prenatal care in an ambulatory setting. These skills include auscultating the fetal heart, measuring symphysis fundal height, and counselling skills. Counselling topics are vast, including genetic screening, changes to diet, exercise routines in pregnancy, and addressing perinatal mood. Many of the topics may be new to the learner, leading to numerous learning opportunities.

To optimize these opportunities, there are several ways to enhance the learning environment.

How to Prepare the Office for Learners

PREPARE THE STAFF AND PATIENTS

Several steps can be taken to streamline the office routines to accommodate learners and make an ambulatory setting more conducive to teaching perinatal care:

- Full collaboration from all members (administrative staff, learners, teachers, and patients) in the teaching environment facilitates the successful integration of teaching (Dent, 2005).
- Patients should be made aware that learners may be involved in their care and be given the opportunity to provide or deny consent (Sprake, 2008).
- Learners can help the integration run smoothly by completing training regarding office procedures, electronic medical record keeping, and other relevant topics (Regan-Smith, 2002).
- Staff should be aware of the clinic's focus on teaching and the differing levels of learners' training when booking patients. This will help make the environment more receptive, removing the pressures of time constraints and allowing for the thoughtful use of space (Dent, 2013).

ARRANGE OFFICE BOOKINGS TO ALLOW TIME FOR TEACHING

Accommodating learners into a busy schedule can be challenging. When a teacher is working alone, they might book between 5 and 15 minutes per patient. This results in a high volume of patients per clinic. In this setting, it may be tempting to have early learners observe in order to see this number of patients. However, learners tend to appreciate and gain more from personally completing the assessments, based on their level of learning (Oberhelman, 2020). To accommodate the learner's pace in the ambulatory setting, the office staff should ensure patients are booked at appropriate time intervals. The office staff should be aware of differing templates based on the individual learner's level and different teaching strategies that may be employed (Fields, 2000). There are several different scheduling models that may be applied.

These include . . .

- Wave scheduling: This scheduling model (Fig. 1) builds in preceptor teaching time without decreasing volume because two patients are seen at the same time (Ferenchik, 1997).
- Purposeful gaps: In this model, time is booked into the schedule or longer appointments are allotted to each patient visit to make sure teaching is timely and not left to chance (Sprake, 2008). The length of time is based on the learner's level of training.
- Catch-up period: Time is allotted at the end of a half day or after three or four patient encounters to review the patients and allow for teaching (Sprake, 2008).

Overall booking schedules will depend on how much time the teacher plans to spend with the learner. Optimal booking should reflect the student's clinical abilities and personalize learning to their level where possible (Fields, 2000).

Time	Learner	Teacher
0900	Sees patient A	Sees patient B
0915	Learner and teacher review patient A	
0930	Learner charts	Sees patient C
0945	Sees patient D	Sees patient E
1000	Learner and teacher review patient D	
1015	Learner charts	Sees patient F

FIGURE 1: SAMPLE "WAVE SCHEDULE."

DEDICATE A SPACE FOR TEACHING AND REVIEWING CASES IN THE CLINIC'S LAYOUT

The environment of an office itself can help facilitate learning. Try to incorporate the learner's perspective on what would help their workflow and learning (Irby, 1995).

The following is a list of equipment and information that may enhance a learning environment:

- Two or more clinic rooms
- Extra chairs in clinic rooms for both staff and learners
- An area for confidential case review
- Access for the learner to the office's electronic medical records
- A desk for the learner to work at
- A secure place for the learner's personal belongings
- Additional perinatal care supplies for learners such as extra fetal dopplers, tape measures, blood pressure cuffs, urine dipsticks, and scales

USE SIGNAGE TO INDICATE THAT THE CLINIC INCLUDES LEARNERS

Consider putting up signs and sending brochures or mass emails that alert patients that learners may be involved in their care. For example, a sign at the clinic entrance may read:

> *WELCOME TO OUR CLINIC*
> *THIS IS A TEACHING CLINIC AFFILIATED WITH UNIVERSITY X*
> *PLEASE NOTE A LEARNER MAY BE INVOLVED IN YOUR CARE*
> *THIS IS AN INCLUSIVE ENVIRONMENT*

The goal is two-fold:

1. Alerts patients of the learning environment
2. Ensures learners know they are expected and welcome

Consider signage alerting patients to the inclusive environment in the office. It may be hard to mitigate some patients' cultural biases, but it is important for teachers to be examples of inclusivity (Kostov, 2018). Most patients appreciate being part of a learning team. Patients from ambulatory care settings report they enjoy giving back and feeling that their experiences can benefit future health professionals and provide new insights (Spencer, 2000; Walters, 2003).

Prenatal Care Models

There are two models to consider when deciding how to incorporate prenatal care into the clinic setting:

1. A dedicated prenatal clinic
2. Prenatal visits integrated into comprehensive care clinics

DEDICATED PRENATAL CLINIC

There are both advantages and limitations to a dedicated prenatal clinic.

The advantages include . . .

- Being able to provide a predictable clinical focus for the learner that appeals to learners at all levels and allows them to build confidence and autonomy
- Being able to include other healthcare professionals, such as a dedicated nurse, lactation consultant, or midwife
- Encouraging knowledge acquisition through repetition

The limitations include . . .

- The need to train office staff to navigate booking and scheduling
- Limited flexibility for patients who are unable to attend appointments on set clinic days
- Non-prenatal patients who need to be fit in for urgent assessment may disrupt the prenatal clinic schedule

Example:

You are paired with a first-year family medicine resident for a morning-dedicated prenatal clinic. The plan for the morning is to see twelve to fifteen prenatal patients of different gestational ages. Before starting the clinic, you review the upcoming patient list to identify the patients the resident will see and the common questions and concerns that each patient may have. You complete the clinic and ask the resident to reflect on his experience that morning. He reports that the repetition of questions and tasks—including measuring symphysis fundal height and auscultation of fetal heart— solidified his learning.

INTEGRATED CLINIC

There are advantages and limitations to an integrated clinic.

The advantages include . . .

- The reinforcement of the idea that low-risk perinatal care can be provided seamlessly within a family medicine clinic and is part of a family doctor's scope of practice
- Prenatal patients may bring other family members for concurrent assessment
- The learner may have previously met the patient for a non-pregnancy-related concern
- The learner can continue to acquire knowledge in other areas

The limitations include . . .

- The need for learners to pivot from managing a variety of other patient concerns to managing prenatal care
- Fewer opportunities for repetition of tasks and knowledge acquisition about prenatal care, as non-obstetrical patients are interspersed between appointments with obstetrical patients

Example:

A second-year family medicine resident is paired with you in a longitudinal clinic in which all family medicine patients might be seen. The resident recognizes one of the patients on the schedule who is being provided with prenatal care. He notes that he has already seen this patient in-clinic before she was pregnant for depressed mood. The resident feels comfortable assessing this patient and asking how her mood has changed since her last visit now that she is pregnant.

TEACHING STRATEGIES TO USE IN PRENATAL CARE

There are six teaching strategies that may be applied independently or used together when teaching prenatal care in an ambulatory care setting:

1. Role-modelling
2. Direct observation
3. Hands-on teaching
4. Huddle
5. Case discussion/presentation
6. Case review

ROLE-MODELLING

Role-modelling is a specific form of learning wherein learning is facilitated by the teacher being the example (Lazarus, 2016). For example, learners can observe teachers using familiar approaches for educating patients at prenatal visits. Typically, role-modelling is used to facilitate learning skills and competencies, including problem-solving, professionalism, and knowing how to think clinically and interact with patients (Irby, 1995).

The advantages of role-modelling are . . .

- Aiding in learners' integration of patient care and professional identity
- Helping learners become more comfortable answering patient questions (Fields, 2000)

The limitations of role-modelling are . . .

- Some learners absorb new knowledge better by actively participating rather than by observing
- The learner and teacher may not be on the same wavelength, which can interfere with learning

Example:

A senior medical student is scheduled to see a thirty-four-year-old pregnant patient in her first trimester of pregnancy. The student is new to prenatal care and although she has heard of prenatal genetic screening and knows the science behind it, she has never explained it to a patient. You offer to model how to do it. The learner watches you counsel the patient during the interaction. One week later, you are paired with the same learner and another patient at 8 weeks gestation is scheduled. This time the learner feels comfortable providing genetic counselling herself.

DIRECT OBSERVATION

Direct observation of the learner can be done in the following ways:

- The teacher sits in for the encounter with the learner
- One-way mirrors are employed to supervise the encounter in real time
- Video recording equipment is used to review the encounter in real time or later

The teacher decides on the method of observation based on several factors, including . . .

- The learner's level of preparation before the clinic
- The complexity of the encounter
- The clinic's setup
- Any other competing clinical demands that may be involved

Before the encounter, the teacher and learner must decide how the learner will contact the teacher when ready to review. Some options include . . .

- Immediate contact through text, mobile phone, intercom or the electronic medical record's instant messaging function
- The teacher entering the patient room at a pre-arranged time while the patient is still present
- The learner exiting the patient room and finding the teacher to review the encounter

Direct observation which includes a one way mirror, video observation or sitting in the room with the patient and learner can be an effective method to conduct a teaching encounter. It allows the teacher to jump in and be hands-on if the situation warrants.

The advantages of direct observation are . . .

- The learner can provide support with care instead of simply observing (Soones, 2015)
- The patient's safety is ensured
- The learner gains confidence by being active in providing care
- The teacher can provide specific feedback based on their observation of the encounter (Rubenstein & Talbot, 2013)

The limitations of direct observation are . . .

- The clinic's pace is slowed because the teacher can observe only one learner at a time
- When the teacher sits in, the patient may bypass the learner and speak directly to the teacher

Example:

A new first-year family medicine resident is scheduled to see a twenty-one-year-old patient for her prenatal physical at twelve weeks gestation. He is new to early pregnancy care. You are the community preceptor, and you decide to stand in the corner to directly observe the interaction. The learner introduces himself and begins. He is quickly overwhelmed by the questions the patient poses, including optimal diet choices in pregnancy, the role of exercise, and so forth. You recognize the learner is flustered and you jump in to answer the questions. Following the questions, you encourage the learner to proceed with the examination, but he is unable to auscultate the fetal heart rate. You demonstrate to the learner how to find the fetal heart.

HANDS-ON TEACHING

Hands-on teaching is a commonly used technique and can be particularly useful for junior learners. In some instances, the teacher will share their findings with the learner to help guide them. Alternatively, both learner and teacher can compare findings after an exam.

The advantage of hands-on teaching is . . .

- The repetition of skills can help learners solidify their examination skills

The limitations of hands-on teaching are . . .

- Some patients are unwilling to have certain components of the physical exam repeated
- It can slow clinic pace, as it requires the teacher to repeat these components

Example:

You are working with a third-year medical student who you have assigned to see a twenty-eight-year-old G2P1 patient at thirty-six-weeks gestation. Before the patient encounter, the learner verbally describes to you how she would measure the symphysis fundal height (SFH). You encourage the learner to measure it on her own and report back. She comes into the reviewing room and reports the SFH is 22 centimetres. Alarmed at the potential stall in growth, you return with the learner to the patient's room to re-measure. You are reassured that the re-measurement is consistent with dates. You take this opportunity to point out the precise landmarks to the learner and the patient. Taking the learner's hand in yours, you examine the landmarks together.

HUDDLE OR PRIMING BEFORE THE START OF A CLINIC

The predictable nature of prenatal care allows for teaching *before* the encounter. The priming method allows the teacher to focus the learner on what they are likely to encounter in the upcoming patient visit (Heidenreich, 2000). This option encourages learners to think about what may be typical at each stage in the pregnancy journey.

The advantages of priming are . . .

- Allowing the learner to see patients alongside the teacher, thus allowing for the more efficient management of patient visits (McGee, 1997)
- Better prepared learners inspire more confidence in patients

The limitations of priming are . . .

- The requirement of predetermined meeting times for the learner and teacher to huddle prior to the start of clinic

- Not every topic can be predicted before seeing the patient, potentially leaving the learner unprepared

Example:

A midwifery student is scheduled to see a patient 6 weeks post-delivery. The patient had an uncomplicated delivery and has not advised the clinic of any particular concerns prior to the appointment. Preceding the start of clinic, you huddle and review the usual topics that need to be reviewed in a postpartum visit, including mood, breastfeeding, lochia, contraceptive options, and future pregnancy counselling. Following the huddle, the learner feels more prepared to counsel the patient on her own.

CASE DISCUSSION

The term "case discussion" refers to a brief review typically done after each patient is seen and while the patient is waiting (Rubenstein & Talbot, 2013). This is the most common form of supervision at most teaching sites. The review can be done either in front of the patient or in a private location. If not done in the patient's presence, the learner and sometimes the teacher return to the patient to conclude the encounter afterwards.

The advantages of case discussion are . . .

- The teacher's ability to review patients in a timely manner with the learner and address any potential urgent situations or time-sensitive tests that may arise during the visit
- The teacher's ability to reassure the learner that their conclusions regarding symptom presentation are accurate
- The learner's ability to reassure patients that the staff physician is fully aware of what occurred at the visit
- Increased opportunities for teaching
- If the brief review is done in front of the patient, the patient can provide the learner with feedback (Regan-Smith, 2002)

The limitations of case discussion are . . .

- Patients may have to wait while their case is being reviewed by the teacher

- The need to review each patient may slow clinic efficiency
- The time for education regarding each case may be limited (Ferenchik, 1997)

Example:

A thirty-eight-week GA patient is scheduled to be seen by a first-year family medicine resident of yours. Prior to the patient arriving, you review the case together and notice a trending increase in the patient's blood pressure during her pregnancy. The learner sees the patient, measures their blood pressure, which remains elevated, and completes the rest of the prenatal visit. He then comes to review the visit with you, while the patient waits in the room. Based on your case discussion, the learner returns to the room and provides the patient with a lab requisition to investigate potential causes for the elevated blood pressure. He had not included lab work in his initial management plan, but you are able to change this after your discussion.

CASE REVIEW

In a case review, the learner reviews a group of patients together, typically at the end of clinic (Rubenstein & Talbot, 2013). This type of review allows learners more time to synthesize salient points (McGee, 1997). This type of teaching may be most beneficial for a senior learner with a good understanding of prenatal care.

The advantages of case reviews are . . .

- They increase the learner's autonomy
- They build the learner's capacity to see a greater number of patients more efficiently, as they will not need to stop to speak to a preceptor after every visit

The limitations of case reviews are . . .

- The decreased face time the learner has with the teacher for each patient
- The possibility of missing important details in the history, physical or investigations resulting in the patient having to return to clinic if they left prior to the case review

Example:

You are paired with a learner, who is in her last 6 months of residency, for a dedicated prenatal clinic. You have worked with her previously. She hopes to increase her autonomy. Prior to the clinic start, you huddle with her to review the morning's list of patients. During this clinic, she will be seeing patients at 12, 16, 20, and 32 weeks' gestation. At the end of clinic, you sit down to review the patients who were seen to determine if the resident has ordered appropriate testing and to confirm that she created and discussed appropriate management plans with the patients. She tells you she appreciated having autonomy during the clinic.

OTHER CONSIDERATIONS

Finally, a reference document outlining important elements of the antenatal visit can be beneficial for the learner to keep organized.

This easily accessible one-page reference document may include . . .

- The typical frequency of visits as the pregnancy progresses
- The elements of care or counselling required at each stage of the pregnancy

This outline is not a step-by-step template. Instead, it can serve as a guide to why testing is done at certain times during a pregnancy and when the next visit should be scheduled in each case. This guide may help learners focus on what they need to remember at each visit to conduct the visit in a timely manner. Finally, it can act as a safety net for senior learners looking to increase their autonomy.

Conclusion

This chapter has provided strategies to ensure that the learner receives valuable experiential learning and that patients receive consistent, thoughtful, and thorough prenatal care. Clinics should be both prepared and flexible enough to accommodate these goals.

REFERENCES

Dent, J. (2013). Learning in ambulatory care. In K. Walsh (Ed.), Oxford textbook of medical education (Chapter 19). Oxford: Oxford University Press.

Dent, J.A. (2005). AMEE guide no 26: clinical teaching in ambulatory care settings: making the most of learning opportunities with outpatients. Medical Teacher, 27(4), 302–315.

Ferenchick, G., Simpson, D., Blackman, J., DaRosa, D., & Dunnington, G. (1997). Strategies for efficient and effective teaching in the ambulatory care setting. Academic Medicine, 72(4), 277-280.

Fields, S., Usatine, R., & Steiner, E. (2000). Teaching medical students in the ambulatory setting. Journal of American Medical Association, 283(18), 2362-4.

Heidenreich, C., Lye, P., Simpson, D., & Lourich, M. (2000). The search for effective and efficient ambulatory teaching methods through the literature. Pediatrics, 105, 231-7.

Irby, D.M. (1995). Teaching and learning in ambulatory care settings: A thematic review of the literature. Academic Medicine, 70(10), 898-931.

Kostov, S., Koppula, S., & Bebenko, O. (2018). Gender differences in women's health and maternity care training: A scoping review. Medical Education Publish 1-9. https://doi.org/10.15694/mep.2018.0000050.1

Lazarus, J. (2016). Precepting 101: Teaching strategies and tips for success for preceptors. Journal of Midwifery & Womens' Health, 61:S11–S21. doi:10.1111/jmwh.12520.

McGee, S.R., & Irby, D.M. (1997). Teaching in the outpatient clinic: practical tips. Journal of General Internal Medicine, 12(S2), S34-S40.

Oberhelman, S., Boswell, C., Jensen, T., Swartz, D., Bruhl, E., O'Brien, M., & Angstman, K. (2020). Student experiences and satisfaction with a novel clerkship patient scheduling. Medical Education Online, 25, 1-9. https://doi.org/10.1080/10872981.2020.1742963

Regan-Smith, M., Young, W.W. & Keller, A.M. (2002). An efficient and effective teaching model for ambulatory education. Academic Medicine, 77(7), 593-599S.

Rubenstein, W., & Talbot, Y. (2013). Medical Teaching in Ambulatory Care (3rd ed.). Toronto: University of Toronto Press.

Soones, T.N., O'Brien, B.C., & Julian, K.A. (2015). Internal medicine residents' perceptions of team-Based Care and its educational value in the continuity clinic: A qualitative study. Journal of General Internal Medicine, 30(9), 1279–85. doi:10.1007/s11606-015-3228

Spencer, J., Blackmore, D., Heard, S., McCrorie, P., McHaffie, D., Scherpbier, A., Gupta, T.S., Singh, K., & Southgate, L. (2000). Patient-oriented learning: a review of the role of the patient in the education of medical students. Medical Education, 34, 851- 857.

Sprake, C., Cantillon, P., Metcalf, J., & Spencer, J. (2008). Teaching in an ambulatory care setting. British Medical Journal, 337:a1156. doi:10.1136/bmj.a1156

Walters, K., Buszewicz, M., Russell, J., & Humphrey, C., (2003). Teaching as therapy: cross sectional and qualitative evaluation of patient's experiences of undergraduate teaching in the community. British Medical Journal, 326, 740-745.

Chapter 2

VIRTUAL PERINATAL CARE: IMPLICATIONS FOR TEACHING

Tali Bogler

Dr. Sonia Jimenez works in an academic family health team. She is in her first 5 years as staff and has incorporated perinatal care into her practice. Over the last few years, Dr. Jimenez has worked on building up her practice and her teaching skills, including supervision of undergraduate and graduate learners. When the COVID–19 pandemic hit, she and her colleagues were required to quickly pivot to virtual care. Dr. Jimenez has no formal training in virtual care teaching and is struggling with the transition to teaching in this new milieu, particularly with regards to virtual prenatal care. She decides to search for articles to learn more about the basic principles of virtual care applied in the prenatal setting, as well as how to teach this topic virtually. Dr. Jimenez finds she needs to clarify the definition, advantages, and disadvantages of virtual prenatal care.

Virtual care is defined as "Any interaction between patients and/or members of their circle of care, occurring remotely (any care that is not delivered in-person) using any forms of communication or information technologies with the aim of facilitating or maximizing the quality and effectiveness of patient care" (Shaw et al., 2018).

The Canadian Medical Association's Virtual Care Playbook (Dermer, 2020) reviews how to provide safe, effective, and efficient virtual care, including how to fit virtual care into practice workflow and technology requirements.

In general, virtual *prenatal* care is some form of combination of in-person and virtual prenatal visits, depending on the patient's needs and medical issues. A responsible care provider must assess whether the pregnant patient is a candidate for virtual care at each visit. A sample prenatal visit schedule that blends in-person and virtual prenatal care is available (Bogler & Bogler, 2020).

Advantages of virtual care *in general* include . . .

1. Limiting patient and provider exposure to COVID–19 and other viruses
2. Avoiding the cost of transit and lost productivity for patients
3. Improving access to care, particularly for individuals with mobility issues, childcare demands, multiple jobs or irregular work hours, or those under quarantine or self-isolation
4. Viewing the patient in their home environment
5. Increased access to care through audio-only virtual prenatal visits (i.e., telephone visits), as opposed to video visits, for those with limited resources

Considerations specific to virtual *prenatal* care include . . .

1. Many patients prefer a blended model of in-person and virtual prenatal visits (Holcomb et al., 2020; Peahr et al., 2020)
2. Many patients are open to virtual care and familiar with home monitoring equipment including a scale and home blood pressure cuff to conduct this type of visit. (e.g., weight and blood pressure)
3. Equivalent outcomes when compared to traditional in-person prenatal care (Butler et al., 2019; Duryea et al., 2021; Palmer et al., 2021)

Disadvantages of virtual care *in general* include . . .

1. The potential for misdiagnosis due to the lack of a physical exam or objective measurement
2. The risk of over-testing to compensate for the absence of physical examination
3. The unequal accessibility of virtual care, particularly when it comes to video platforms, which can worsen existing healthcare inequities (e.g., patients unable to communicate in the same language as their

provider or lacking the necessary digital literacy, computer access, and/ or Internet)

4. The possibility of missing patients' non-verbal emotional cues pertaining to mental health when using audio only

5. Adding an additional layer between patient and provider, making it more difficult to build rapport, particularly with audio-only virtual visits

Considerations specific to virtual *prenatal* care include . . .

1. A lack of reassurance (for both patient and provider) from hearing a fetal heartbeat

2. The possibility of inadequate screening for intimate partner violence (IPV), as telephone lines may not be confidential, or the patient may struggle to access a private space. Pregnancy is a high-risk time for IPV (Long et al., 2019), which also increases during stay-at-home and lockdown orders

3. Challenges to the healthcare provider's ability to accurately screen for perinatal mood and anxiety disorders (PMADS)

After reflecting on the advantages, disadvantages, and safety considerations of virtual prenatal care, Dr. Jimenez decides to look for articles on how to go about teaching and supervising virtual care, including prenatal care. Unfortunately, she does not find any literature on teaching virtual prenatal care specifically; however, she does find a few excellent resources on teaching virtual care and hopes to apply some of these principles to her teaching in this area in particular.

Eight Tips for Supervising Learners Providing Virtual Prenatal Care

This section will expand on the following eight tips for supervising learners providing virtual prenatal care:

1. Ask about the learner's experience with virtual care
2. Determine the level of supervision they need
3. Select the technological tool best suited to the situation
4. Consider your supervision approach

5. Ensure the learner obtains patient consent
6. Review the patient's presentation in the context of virtual care
7. Review the learner's documentation of their visit
8. Provide evaluation and consider providing an evaluation note

ASK ABOUT THE LEARNER'S EXPERIENCE WITH VIRTUAL CARE

Consider asking the learner the following questions:

- How much experience have you had with virtual prenatal care? Learners will likely have varied experiences with virtual care, including digital technologies and tools.
- Are you comfortable with the platform we are using in this office?
- Are you aware of the limitations that are inherent to virtual prenatal care?

DETERMINE THE LEVEL OF SUPERVISION REQUIRED BY THE LEARNER FOR VIRTUAL CARE

The teacher should consider the following:

- Their previous experience with the learner
- The learner's previous experience with prenatal care in general and with virtual prenatal care in specific
- The learner's clinical skills and personal attributes

Example:

You have been working with a 4th-year clinical clerk who is planning on pursuing a surgical residency. You have observed that this learner has particularly strong procedural and physical examination skills, requiring minimal supervision for these encounters. However, at times, he rushes through history taking and misses pertinent psychosocial components. The learner is scheduled to do a virtual prenatal visit with a pregnant patient who is experiencing anxiety during the second trimester. You decide to ask the learner to do a three-way-call so you can listen in on the conversation and provide more direct supervision for the encounter.

SELECT THE TECHNOLOGICAL TOOL APPROPRIATE FOR THE SITUATION

The teacher should decide whether to use a video platform versus telephone based on the following:

1. Which tools are available in the clinical environment to practice virtual care
2. Level of comfort of the patient, learner, and teacher with the various technological modalities
3. The privacy and confidentiality of the chosen platform

The modality might change between patients, as each of their technological literacy, comfort, and access will differ.

Example:

You are working with a 1st-year family medicine resident who gained a lot of experience with virtual care during her previous rotation, specifically using video modalities such as Zoom for Healthcare. This learner has a telephone virtual prenatal appointment booked with a patient of yours that is a newcomer to Canada and is financially disadvantaged. The learner worries about using "low tech" methods for prenatal care, such as the telephone. You tell her that for this patient, given possible barriers, including a lack of access to a private computer, it would be best to start by using the telephone as the technological tool of choice.

CONSIDER YOUR SUPERVISION APPROACH

It can be helpful to stratify supervision approaches for virtual care based on whether the teacher and learner are in the same location and how much supervision is required.

If the teacher and learner are in the same location

If more supervision is required . . .

- The teacher can sit in the same room for the encounter while the patient is on speaker phone or video call

If less supervision is required . . .

- The teacher and learner can decide ahead of time the best way to review cases, taking into consideration whether there are other learners in the clinic or other competing demands for the teacher's time
- After the learner completes the initial virtual encounter with the patient, the learner can review the case with the teacher in the following ways:
  - Between cases: The patient is either put on hold or told they will be called back once the case is reviewed
  - At the end of the clinic: All cases are reviewed, and the patients are told they will be called back if there is any change in management. The teacher may join the call with the patient on speaker phone to discuss the diagnosis and plan.

If the teacher and learner are not in the same location (i.e., remote supervision)

There are different video modalities that can be employed for remote supervision. Zoom videoconferencing software can be helpful when supervising learners. This platform allows an online waiting room (the clinical waiting room), a main session (the teaching room), and multiple breakout rooms (clinic rooms) (Domb et al., 2021). The teacher can move from one breakout room to another, observing clinical encounters in real time.

If more supervision is required . . .

- The teacher, learner, and patient can make a three-way telephone or video call, so that the teacher can listen to or watch the visit directly

If less supervision is required . . .

- After the learner completes the initial virtual encounter with the patient, the learner can review the case with the teacher either between cases or at the end of the clinic (as described in the previous section)

Regardless of the review process undertaken, it is important to arrange easy options for the learner to access the teacher for impromptu discussions as needed (e.g., via text or phone calls).

Example:

You are supervising a senior obstetrics resident remotely today. You are both scheduled to see patients simultaneously. You discuss with the learner before the clinic begins the review process and easy options for impromptu questions. Since you will be using your main phone to call patients yourself, you also provide the resident with an alternate phone number that he can call when he needs or advise him to use instant messaging through the electronic medical record.

ENSURE THE LEARNER OBTAINS PATIENT CONSENT TO PROVIDE VIRTUAL CARE

Whichever technology is decided on, it is important for the learner to understand its limitations and legal requirements before using it for patient care. Consider having a script that providers and learners can use at the start of a virtual patient encounter. There is an example at end of this chapter.

ENSURE THE LEARNER KNOWS HOW TO ASSESS IF A VIRTUAL CARE VISIT IS APPROPRIATE

The teacher should ensure the learner considers the following:

1. Does the patient have the equipment clinically necessary for that particular virtual visit (e.g., blood pressure cuff and scale)?
2. Do they have a confidential space to engage in the visit?
3. Are they comfortable with virtual care?

Example:

You ask a new family medicine resident to conduct a virtual prenatal visit for a pregnant patient of yours who is at 30 weeks gestation. When the learner reviews the case, she reports that the patient did not have a blood pressure machine at home. During the visit, the patient endorsed having headaches intermittently throughout the pregnancy, which had worsened over the last 2 weeks. The learner scheduled a follow-up visit at 32 weeks gestation. Together, you call the patient back to offer an in-person assessment later that afternoon to measure the blood pressure and conduct a physical examination to rule out preeclampsia.

REVIEW THE LEARNER'S DOCUMENTATION OF THEIR VISIT

Consider the following:

- An important part of the virtual visit is documenting that informed verbal consent was obtained at the beginning of the medical note. See the end of this chapter for a template to use for documentation purposes. A template could also be created for an electronic medical record, which can be shown to the learner in advance of their first patient interaction.
- The learner must understand that follow-up appointments and investigations need to be clearly documented and easy to operationalize, particularly with virtual prenatal care

PROVIDE EVALUATION AND CONSIDER PROVIDING AN EVALUATION NOTE

Even though the prenatal visit is virtual, the teacher should remember to provide feedback, as in any teaching session. It is important to leave time for learner feedback, whether in-person or virtual. For further details on evaluation, please see Chapter 10.

Example:

You are remotely supervising two learners in a virtual clinic. You block off 30 minutes at the end of the clinic to elicit feedback from the learners, including their successes and challenges with remote learning. You plan to incorporate their feedback into the next time you supervise learners virtually.

Into the Future

Virtual care will likely be part of patient care moving forward. As a result, it is imperative to find a robust way to ensure learners are provided successful educational opportunities in virtual prenatal care. This includes enabling faculty to observe and evaluate encounters, thereby providing patients with a safe and effective platform through which to receive virtual prenatal care in the teaching setting.

Sample Script for Obtaining Consent Prior to Proceeding with Virtual Care

Just like online shopping or email, virtual care has some inherent privacy and security risks that your health information may be intercepted or unintentionally disclosed. We want to make sure you understand this before we proceed. In order to improve privacy and confidentiality, you should also take steps to participate in this virtual care encounter in a private setting and should not use an employer's or someone else's device, as they may be able to access your information.

If you want more information, please check the link on our (website/confirmation email/etc.). If it is determined that you require a physical exam, you may need to be assessed in person. You should also understand that virtual care is not a substitute for visiting the emergency department if urgent care is needed. Are you OK to continue?

Template for Documenting Consent Obtained for Virtual Care

Informed verbal consent was obtained from this patient to communicate and provide care using virtual and other telecommunications tools. This patient has been explained the risks related to unauthorized disclosure or interception of personal health information and steps they can take to help protect their information. We have discussed that care provided through video or audio communication cannot replace the need for physical examination or an in-person visit for some disorders or urgent problems, and the patient understands the need to seek urgent care in an emergency department as necessary.

Both templates above are from the following website:

https://www.afhto.ca/sites/default/files/2020-03/Virtual%20Care%20Patient%20Consent%20FAQ.pdf

REFERENCES

Bogler, T., & Bogler, O. (2020). Interim schedule for pregnant women and children during the COVID–19 pandemic. Canadian Family Physician, 66(5):e155-e161.

Butler-Tobah, Y.S., LeBlanc, A., & Branda, M.E. (2019). Randomized comparison of a reduced-visit prenatal care model enhanced with remote monitoring. American Journal of Obstetrics and Gynecology, 221(6), e631-638.

Dermer, M. Canadian Medical Association CoFPoC, Royal College of Physicians and Surgeons of Canada. Virtual care playbook. Canadian Medical Association Web site. https://www.cma.ca/sites/default/files/ pdf/Virtual-Care-Playbook_mar2020_E.pdf. Updated March 2020.

Domb, S., Manly, E., & Elman, D. (2021). Pandemic patch-up: Using Zoom videoconferencing software to create a virtual teaching clinic. Canadian Family Physician, 67(1), 65-68.

Duryea, E.L., Adhikari, E.H., Ambia, A., Spong, C., McIntire, D., & Nelson, D.B. (2021). Comparison between in-person and audio-only virtual prenatal visits and perinatal outcomes. Journal of the American Medical Association Network Open, 4(4), e215854.

Holcomb, D., Faucher, M.A., Bouzid, J., Quint-Bouzid, M., Nelson, D.B., & Duryea, E. (2020). Patient perspectives on audio-only virtual prenatal visits amidst the severe acute respiratory syndrome. Coronavirus 2 (SARS-CoV-2) Pandemic. Obstetrics and Gynecology, 136(2), 317-322.

Long, A.J., Golfar, A., & Olson, D.M. (2019). Screening in the prenatal period for intimate partner violence and history of abuse: A survey of Edmonton obstetrician/gynaecologists. Canadian Journal of Obstetrics and Gynecology, 41(1), 38-45.

Ontario MD Virtual Care, (2020). https://ontariomd.vc/how-can-i-start-using-virtual-care-2/

Palmer, K.R., Tanner, M., & Davies-Tuck, M. (2021). Widespread implementation of a low-cost telehealth service in the delivery of antenatal care during the COVID-19 pandemic: an interrupted time-series analysis. Lancet, 398(10294), 41-52.

Peahl, A.F., Novara, A., Heisler, M., Dalton, V.K., Moniz, M.H., & Smith, R.D. (2020). Patient preferences for prenatal and postpartum care delivery: A survey of postpartum women. Obstetrics and Gynecology, 135(5), 1038-1046.

Shaw, J., Jamieson, T., Agarwal, P., Griffin, B., Wong, I., & Bhatia, R.S. (2018). Virtual care policy recommendations for patient-centred primary care: findings of a consensus policy dialogue using a nominal group technique. Journal of Telemedicine and Telecare, 24(9), 608-615.

United Nations. UN News website. UN chief calls for domestic violence "ceasefire" amid "horrifying global surge." April 6 A, 2021. https://news.un.org/en/story/2020/04/1061052.

Chapter 3

TEACHING LEARNERS DURING
LABOUR AND BIRTH

ANNE BIRINGER, MILENA FORTE

Dr. Meseret Berhane is a new member of your family medicine perinatal call group who recently completed her extra training in perinatal care. To date, her only clinical experience at your hospital has been doing the observed deliveries as required for privileges. Your team always has a resident working with the staff physician. Meseret is anxious about her first day on call at the hospital as she has not had much experience working with residents. She is keen to learn some teaching strategies to use during shifts while she also hones her own skills. The following chapter summarizes some of the tips she learns when shadowing her colleagues.

The teaching of intrapartum care provides an opportunity for learners to have one-on-one supervision for an extended period of time in a variety of situations. Bedside teaching fosters the acquisition of clinical skills and the development of empathy, as well as instills confidence and builds up the doctor-patient relationship (Carty et al., 2020). The skills acquired can be applied in multiple settings—not just labour and delivery. The supervisor will have the opportunity to observe the resident's clinical competence, communication skills, and their ability to collaborate with the team and handle emergencies while they triage and prioritize patient care.

In addition to providing multiple clinical teaching opportunities, intrapartum care is a time for learners to see their teachers as role models in action, modelling clinical competency, full scope care, their role in the hospital, teamwork, and continuity of care. This is particularly important for the family medicine learner who is considering including intrapartum care in their future. However, all learners can benefit from this experience. Successful family medicine perinatal care education programs have highly visible, strong family medicine role models who . . .

- Are competent preceptors
- Model passion for and enjoyment of family medicine perinatal care
- Model sustainable practice and work-life balance (Biringer et al., 2018)

The experience of providing clinical care during one of the most momentous events in a patient's life adds to its intensity for both learner and teacher. The skills learned in this setting can have much broader applications than perinatal care. This chapter will review strategies for clinical teaching of intrapartum perinatal care skills.

Considerations in Bedside Teaching of Intrapartum Care

There is no substitute for learning from patients. Simulation has an important role in skills training but can never fully replace the complexity and nuances of being at the bedside. As a learner, there is much to be gleaned by observing and participating in someone's care in real time. Childbirth is one of the most intense and momentous experiences of a person's life and can present many teachable moments. However, it can also be daunting for the patient, learner, and teacher.

The following section explores some opportunities and challenges for bedside teaching. It is helpful to consider some of these issues with regards to the patient, the learner, the teacher, and the context.

THE PATIENT

In general, patients feel positive about the involvement of learners in their care. Perinatal patients are generally willing to participate in teaching as long as they have the option to provide or decline consent. It is also vital that the learners are respectful and confidentiality is maintained. Patients recognize that they can contribute to learning with their lived experience of labour and birth. However, in general, they will prioritize their own well-being over the learners' experience—a tension teachers will likely encounter (Carty et al., 2020).

Teachers can actively integrate the patient as a direct teacher by asking them to give feedback to the learner in appropriate situations.

Example:

"You seemed uncomfortable with that procedure. Could you tell Dr. Salomon what they could have done to make it less painful?"

By spending time with patients, learners can be a part of the labour and birth journey. This can be a powerful experience that enhances clinical learning. These complex interpersonal and emotional situations can provide a humanizing effect to the practice of medicine (Masters, 2020).

Labour and delivery presents a unique opportunity to spend time with a patient over the course of their care. Despite the fact that technology plays an increasingly large role in monitoring normal as well as complicated labour, it is important that the teacher highlights and models the importance of focusing on the person in labour, not just the computerized medical record and electronic fetal heart tracing.

Example:

When the team enters the room, rather than heading straight to the monitor to examine the "strip," the teacher addresses the patient and their support people before checking on the various machines in the room.

Intimate examinations require exquisite sensitivity at all times, as they can be uncomfortable and can cause harm. However, learners do need to practise this skill to progress. The approach to the patient, communication, and technique can be transferred to pelvic examinations and, in fact, any aspect of the physical examination in any setting.

Consider the following:

- Be particularly sensitive if there is a history of trauma or other psychological or cultural reasons for heightened anxiety during internal examinations (Güneş & Karaçam, 2017)

- Consider avoiding double examinations on patients who are labouring without analgesia if possible
- Avoid unnecessary exams, as the risk of infection, such as chorioamnionitis, increases with the number of vaginal examinations (Gluck et al., 2020)

In teaching internal examination techniques, be sure to do the following:

- Before entering the room, coach the learner to approach the patient with sensitivity and gentleness
- Explain the process to the patient, including the rationale for examining at that particular time
- Obtain consent and ensure privacy
- Tell the learner which aspects of the examination they are expected to describe prior conducting the exam
- Ideally, conduct the examination when the patient has an empty bladder and is between contractions, with the patient using their breathing to relax their muscles

Example:

"I would like you to examine our patient to determine the cervical dilation and station of the fetal head. We will work on position later in the labour. Use lots of lubricant to advance your two fingers, keeping the pressure away from the sensitive structures at the anterior fourchette. Once your fingers reach the cervix, then open them to determine dilation and describe where the leading part of the fetal head is in relation to the ischial spines."

THE LEARNER

Learners bring with them variable levels of interest, prior knowledge, and attitudes toward perinatal care. Many of our current and future learners fall into the generational cohort of Millennials and Gen Z, and as such, may have specific learning styles and preferences (see Chapter 6). Although it is easy to teach the learner who is committed to perinatal care, there are many ways to engage the uninterested learner (see Chapter 8). While they are involved in the intense experience of childbirth, the accomplished teacher can engage these learners with new skills that are applicable to any context.

Some examples of learner-related issues that teachers might encounter include . . .

- **Learners with different learning styles**: Although the concept of learning styles has been debated, the most commonly used model is VARK (visual, auditory, read/write, kinesthetic). The majority of medical learners are multimodal. However, learning in labour and delivery heavily favours those who are comfortable with kinesthetic learning, a learning style in which students learn by carrying out physical activities rather than listening to lectures or watching demonstrations (Hernandez et al., 2020).
- **The anxious learner**: This learner may have a higher-than-expected fear of bad outcomes given the perceived high-stakes nature of intrapartum care.

Example:

You are meeting with a learner on their first day of the perinatal care rotation. You ask about their previous experience with intrapartum care and the learner describes a situation when they were on their pediatric rotation and the team was called stat to resuscitate a baby that was born unexpectedly "flat." The memory of the limp baby and the hysterical parents has convinced the learner that things can go terribly wrong at any time in labour and delivery, and they are very anxious about being a part of it. You acknowledge that this must have been a very traumatic experience for the learner and try to reassure them by stating that the vast majority of patients and their babies do very well. You finish by asking how you can support them throughout this rotation.

In general . . .

- Identify the anxious learner and try to clarify the origins of their anxiety
- Start with the learner observing as the teacher role models
- Gauge the learner's desire or willingness to participate over time, and give them graduated responsibilities

Other learners who may require special attention may include . . .

1. Learners with poor manual dexterity (see the special considerations at the end of this chapter)
2. Male learners who experience challenges being accepted into the perinatal care environment (see the special considerations at the end of this chapter)
3. Multiple learners at different levels and with varied levels of interest. With careful planning, learners at different stages of training can be welcomed into the labour and delivery environment and given tasks commensurate with their skill.

Example:

The more experienced learner might be able to conduct the delivery while the novice student delivers the placenta. A senior obstetrical resident might then repair a third-degree tear under the supervision of their staff.

THE TEACHER

Teachers in perinatal care must balance roles as the most responsible physician for the patient in question and the primary supervisor for the learner on a particular day. At times, this occurs seamlessly, when the case is straightforward or the resident is particularly capable. At other times, the two roles can create tension (Gingerich et al., 2018).

Furthermore, teachers have their own set of values, experiences, and biases that impact how they interact with learners. The following teacher-dependent characteristics may impact teaching (https://www.scholarify.in/factors-affecting-teaching/):

1. Knowledge of the subject
2. Knowledge of the learners
3. Teaching skills (perhaps from reading this book!)
4. Friendliness and approachability

Experienced teachers may feel more comfortable giving learners more autonomy, while new teachers may wish to be more hands-on while they consolidate their own skills. Teachers may self-identify or identify colleagues as more "hands-off" or "hands-on" supervisors. However, all teachers will dynamically shift approaches depending on context (Gingerich et al., 2018).

New teachers have unique challenges. Meseret exemplifies the new teacher, not yet comfortable with her own clinical skills or the new clinical environment, and concerned about the added layer of having a learner. She is just starting to develop her identity as a teacher. However, being close to the learner's level can be an advantage, because the teacher may be very tuned in to their needs. It is important that Meseret be supported in her clinical and academic growth by her colleagues. She needs to ensure that her own clinical skills are secure and should understand that it is acceptable to prioritize her own skill development over learner participation in the beginning. As her comfort with her own skills progresses, she will be able to allow more participation by the learner, depending on their skills and knowledge.

THE CONTEXT

Many contextual factors contribute to the unique challenges of teaching intrapartum care. There is very little predictability to each shift—in terms of clinical activity and acuity of cases. In addition, internal examinations cannot be supervised under direct visualization. Possible approaches to some of these contextual factors are described below.

Volume and Case Mix Is Unpredictable

Teaching opportunities are dependent on activity in labour and delivery. Even over a rotation, the exposure to different situations will not necessarily even out or cover all important scenarios. Here are some strategies to address this issue:

1. Use each situation as an opportunity for broader teaching.

    Examples:
    "You did an excellent job rupturing the membranes. Would you manage labour differently if there had been meconium in the amniotic fluid?"

"Those variable decelerations responded well to maternal repositioning. Can you tell me about the other components of intrauterine resuscitation?"

2. Utilize simulation to practise rare but emergency situations. (See Chapter 4.)

3. Take downtime in labour and delivery as an opportunity to review common case presentations with the learner at a comfortable pace, where they can ask questions without a patient present.

Internal Examinations "Happen in the Dark"

Teachers have to rely on the resident's description of what they are feeling. In addition, there is poor inter-observer agreement as to some components of the cervical exam, such as station of fetal head (Buchmann & Libhaber, 2008). However, learning by feeling, describing, and comparing can be a profound experience for all learners.

Intrapartum Care Can Quickly Turn into a Crisis

Although labour and birth are often medically uneventful, there is always the spectre of a true emergency. This can make both teachers and learners anxious and lead to educational challenges in the acute situation. At times, the intensity of the birth experience may interfere with full involvement of the learner. While it may be appropriate to bypass the learner in a crisis, it is important to debrief thoughtfully with the learner immediately afterwards—and to maintain contact with them over time if there was a bad outcome. These unexpected situations can offer "teachable moments" (Whitman, & Magill, 2000)— unplanned opportunities for the teacher to address the current issue when the learner is very engaged—with resultant meaningful learning.

Specific Strategies

Clinical teaching can be described as happening "backstage"—any preparatory work or debriefing that happens without the patient present, outside the patient room, and "onstage"--anything that happens with the patient present.

This section will address many of the situations that occur during clinical teaching in labour and delivery.

BACKSTAGE (PRIOR TO ENGAGING WITH THE PATIENT)

Preparing the Learning Environment

Pay Attention to Relationships. Particularly for family medicine learners, it is important that the hospital be "family medicine friendly." This requires:

- The presence of adequate number of family physicians
- A robust low-risk program
- Acceptance (both clinical and educational) by the multi-professional team (Biringer et al., 2018)

It is up to both the individual teacher and the educational program to nurture these relationships to ensure a safe and accepting learning environment. It is well known that when the labour and delivery unit is seen as a hostile learning environment, this interferes with learning and patient care (Tobin et al., 2006). Although the individual teacher may not have control over the labour and delivery environment, they can be a role model in interprofessional collaboration and relationship-building and include the learner in all interactions throughout the labour and birth process. When interactions are not ideal, teachers can identify these moments and reflect with the learner on how to optimize the situation, always focusing on the patient as the centre of care. Learners can be involved in formal opportunities for interprofessional collaboration and learning, such as the MORE[OB] (Managing Obstetrical Risk Efficiently) course (https://www. moreob.com). When learners see that their teachers are valued members of the perinatal care team, they are able to see themselves in those roles.

Example:

You are an experienced intrapartum care provider and are very involved in the development of hospital protocols for labour and delivery. You enjoy attending the monthly Labour and Delivery (L and D) Committee meetings and feel that you have developed very good relationships with a number of your interprofessional colleagues. In fact, many of the L and D nurses and physicians and their families have become your patients. They have told you that they respect the relationships that you have with your pregnant and birthing patients.

When you are paired with a learner and there is no patient in labour, you include them in all of your professional activities. The learners have commented on the mutual respect that they observe when you are asking an obstetrician for consultation, and they feel they are somehow swept up into the goodwill that seems to be accorded to you.

Enlist the Interprofessional Team. There is much opportunity for the other members of the perinatal care team (such as nurses, obstetricians, respiratory technologists, or midwives) to become involved as teachers. It is important to set the stage for their involvement. Their role needs to be defined, their expertise acknowledged, and their teaching efforts rewarded, rather than being seen as extra work.

Assemble Teaching Aids. Teachers might consider keeping a "teachers' kit" (see Fig. 1) in a convenient location where they can physically demonstrate and the resident can practise manual skills, such as application of fetal scalp electrode, doing a somersault manoeuvre for a nuchal cord, and so on. This practice ensures that the learner is more comfortable with a particular simulation before embarking on performing the procedure on a patient.

Possible contents for a "Teachers' Kit"

Pelvis and doll with placenta and cord
Suture material and needle driver, towels to sew
Scalp electrode
Amniotomy hook and balloon
Dilation board
Vacuum extractors
Foley catheter and model for insertion

FIGURE 1: POSSIBLE CONTENTS FOR A "TEACHERS' KIT."

Preparing the Patient for Learner Participation

Ideally, all pregnant people will be informed, prior to admission to hospital, that learners will be involved in their intrapartum care. Ensure that the learner's role is discussed during prenatal visits and any concerns are addressed prior to admission. This is particularly important where there are concerns about the participation of male learners or specific patient experiences that require particular attention during intrapartum care. Ideally, these conversations happen when patients first come into care.

Example:

"Congratulations on your first pregnancy. I'm delighted that you have chosen our team to follow your pregnancy and birth. I want to explain how our clinic functions, as this is your first time here. We are a teaching practice affiliated with university X and hospital Y. There will always be learners involved in your care, from your prenatal visits to your hospital stay. These learners may be of any gender and are all closely supervised by the staff physicians. If you have any concerns, please do not hesitate to raise them with me or another supervising doctor."

A strong, pre-existing doctor-patient relationship will benefit teaching in many ways. In situations where the teacher is providing intrapartum care to a patient they have not met before, it is extremely important to set up this relationship from the first moment possible—a skill that is easily role-modelled to learners. However, regardless of the principles about learner involvement that have been discussed and agreed upon during prior visits, it is critical to obtain informed consent at every juncture. Some examples of how to obtain consent in the moment include:

- *"This is Dr. X, one of our family medicine residents. They will be working with me today, and it is important that they and I both be on the same page. Would it be OK with you if we both did a vaginal exam to make sure that we agree on the findings? Would you mind if we discussed our findings together in front of you?"*
- *"We have discussed the risks and benefits of breaking the waters at this point in labour. Is it OK with you if Dr. Y breaks your waters under my supervision?"*

- *"I understand that you would like me to deliver the baby. I can assure you that my hands will be on your baby's head alongside Dr. Z's as they are being born."*

Preparing the Learner

Preparing the learner for procedures with which they may not be comfortable is critical for learner self-confidence. It is also important for patient safety and comfort, as well as their confidence in the learner. It is important to do the following:

1. Clarify their learning goals for that shift/rotation. Given that not all learners will provide intrapartum care in their future careers, encourage all learners to find relevant learning goals for each encounter.

   Example:
   "Based on our discussion this morning and your interest in surgery, I am going to suggest that we focus on your suturing and knot-tying. Please take every opportunity to practise on our suture board during the shift so that we can focus on the perineal repair when we have the opportunity."

2. Identify the learner's previous experiences specific to the procedure at hand. Clarify what they have done independently, where they would like more experience, and what they would prefer to observe.

   Example:
   "I understand that you learned the examination of the newborn as a clinical clerk. Would you like to check this baby under my supervision, or would you prefer to watch me do the first one?"

3. Do a "dry run" of the procedure before entering the patient's room. This involves modelling, simulation, and orientation with regard to the practical aspects of the task at hand.

   Example:
   "Let's review the application of a scalp electrode before we go into the patient's room. I have one in our teaching kit that you can practise with."

ONSTAGE (IN THE ROOM)

Direct Demonstration

It is sometimes more helpful to demonstrate the procedure in detail rather than describing it. This technique can save time and confusion when verbal instructions might be unclear. The rationale for the manoeuvre can be explained to the learner at the same time to solidify their knowledge acquisition.

Some common examples:

- *"Note how I put my hand just above the symphysis pubis and push up against the uterus while I am putting steady traction on the umbilical cord to deliver the placenta. This prevents uterine inversion. Only after the placenta delivers should you put your hand at the top of the fundus to assess uterine tone or massage the uterus."*
- *"I find it easier to mount the needle on the needle driver this way—it gives me more control and is less likely to slip or rotate."*
- *"I put the next stitch in at this spot. It needs to be deep and come out at the midline before taking the same big bite on the other side. It is called the crown stitch and brings the bulbocavernosus muscle together."*

Thinking Out Loud

It is helpful for the learner to "hear" the teacher's thought processes. This needs to be done with attention to what the patient and other team members will also be hearing.

Example:

"The head has been slow to descend (in this second-time mother), which makes me wonder if we are dealing with a larger-than-expected baby." (This explains to the learner why you might be worried or performed a certain task). *"If that is the case, we should all be ready for the possibility that the shoulders might be difficult to deliver. Thus, I want to be prepared with a stool on the side of the baby's back. I also want to enlist the nurse and the partner to potentially help with leg flexion."* (While everyone is waiting, the teacher could also run through the sequential manoeuvres to relieve a shoulder dystocia.)

In the above example, if the learner has internalized the information about shoulder dystocia, they should then be prepared to handle a novel situation. Medical educators are being challenged to train their learners for adaptive expertise. Adaptive expertise refers to the ability to innovate and be creative in new situations in contrast to routine expertise (doing things over and over until they become experts), which focuses on accuracy and efficiency (Lajoie & Gube, 2018). In this situation, using "what if" questions encourages the learner to think about how they would handle novel situations:

"Fortunately for us, this baby delivered after McRoberts manoeuvre. What would you have done if the patient had been pushing on all fours? How would you have managed a shoulder dystocia in that position?"

Teaching to the Room

This refers to explanations that are made in the birthing room to the patient and their supports. The inexperienced learner may not know this information; however, by "teaching to the room," the learner experiences the content in a non-threatening way. No one else knows that this is new information for the learner. You should prepare the learner that this will be happening, as in this example:

"When we go back in to help the patient with the second stage of labour, pay attention to what I am discussing with the patient—you might be able to pick up some tips."

This is a purposeful and deliberate strategy, which role-models communication skills and also teaches content. The teacher and learner must debrief afterward to ensure that the learner received this information and is able to ask questions. Some examples of this interaction are:

- *"We will try several different positions for the second stage of labour until we find one that works for you. Given your situation, you might find a supported squat works the best. Let me show you how to get into that position."*
- *"I can see by your baby's heart rate pattern that she is not tolerating the final stages of the birth process, and I would recommend that we assist you by using the vacuum. Let me explain how that works and the risks to you and the baby."*

Teacher Examines First

The traditional approach to teaching is for the learner to examine first and then report to the teacher. This is then followed by the teacher's examination and verification or explanation for the difference in findings. However, this order does not allow the learner to "try again" and correct their interpretation. Consider the opposite order, with the teacher examining first. Some situations where this is useful include:

- **Cervical dilation, fetal station, and position.** After obtaining patient consent for a double exam, the teacher examines the patient first, without revealing their findings to the learner. Then, while the learner examines the patient, they are encouraged to speak aloud, describing what they feel in terms of dilation, position, and descent. This gives an excellent opportunity to guide the learner if they have described the findings inaccurately. For example:
  - If they missed an anterior lip, they can be directed to palpate anteriorly for a lip of cervix that they did not appreciate.
  - If they misdiagnosed the position, the teacher can explain what makes the occiput and sinciput "feel" different, while the learner still has the opportunity to palpate.
- **Artificial rupture of membranes.** Teacher first ascertains whether it is appropriate and safe to rupture the patient's membranes. After preparing the learner, the teacher is present and able to talk them through the procedure. If they struggle, the teacher can reinforce clinical "tricks" to make the procedure easier, such as positioning the patient with hips on fists, waiting for a contraction, asking an assistant for fundal pressure, and so on.

Hand Over Hand

Nothing can substitute for "hands-on" learning. As it is often difficult to describe the sensation of certain procedures, the teacher might, with the learner's permission, place their hand(s) over the learner's hands to assess and model the amount of pressure or tension that is appropriate. Some situations where this is useful include:

- **Crowning.** The teacher places their hands over the learner's hands during second stage as the head begins to emerge. The teacher can feel the exact moment of crowning and coach the patient to stop pushing, while the learner feels the sensation of crowning with their own hands. In time, they will be able to coach the patient themselves.
- **Delivery of the placenta.** By applying their hands, the teacher will sense if there is too much tension on the cord or not enough countertraction with the other hand, which is "guarding" the uterus.

As the learner becomes more proficient, the teacher may advance the supervision from having both hands applied, to simply poising their hands at the ready and finally, not putting gloves on unless a problem develops (see the section below on graduating responsibility).

Graduating Responsibility Or "Letting Go"

The goal for teachers is to facilitate the learner's journey toward independent practice. In order to do this, teachers need to be able to "let go" when appropriate. This requires that they trust the learner and give them an opportunity to demonstrate their clinical skills with varying levels of support (Ten Cate et al., 2016). How do teachers know when to let go? This will be different for every teacher and each learner, and it is not without some risk. Trusting someone else to provide care to patients can leave teachers feeling vulnerable.

It may not always be appropriate to let go. There are several factors that may help teachers decide when to do so and how. These factors are related to the:

1. Learner
2. Context
3. Teacher-learner relationship
4. Teacher
5. Physician-patient relationship

Learner. Learner factors are important to consider, as teachers need to trust their learners not only to do the right thing, but also to behave predictably and reliably and to seek help when needed. This is particularly important on the labour floor when teachers rely on their learners to manage potentially acute situations. There are many questions the teacher will consider when deciding how much to let go.

Some of these questions have to do with the learner's clinical skills, including . . .

1. What level of training do they have? (Are they in their undergraduate or postgraduate training? What year?)
2. What previous experience do they have in perinatal care?
3. Have they demonstrated competence in prior interactions?
4. Is there information about the learner available that was obtained from other teachers prior to their clinical rotation?

Other questions will have to do with the learner's attributes, including . . .

1. Are they responsible?
2. Do they show motivation?
3. Are they compassionate?
4. Do they demonstrate self-awareness?

Context. The teacher will also have to consider factors that are not specific to the learner but impact their own ability to "let go." These include . . .

1. Their current volume of work
2. The patient's acuity
3. The nature of the task at hand
4. The timing of the visit or interaction (for instance, if it is in the middle of the night or at handover time)
5. The resources available (including the availability of other team members)

Teacher-Learner Relationship. Previous interactions with learners may also influence how comfortable the teacher is letting them take on more responsibility. This may include . . .

1. Whether they have worked together previously in labour and delivery
2. Whether they have worked together in other clinical contexts
3. Whether they have worked together on committees or research projects
4. Whether they have a longitudinal or episodic relationship

Teacher. Some teachers prefer to be more hands-on as oppose to hands-off. A teacher's confidence in letting go may also vary with their own clinical skills in a particular area or their experience as a teacher. It is important to occasionally reflect on one's own teaching style and comfort level over the course of a teaching career.

Physician-Patient Relationship. The physician-patient relationship may influence how involved the teacher chooses to be or how much autonomy they grant the learner. For example, when meeting a patient at the same time (or after) the learner, the teacher may feel less inclined to "take over," as the learner may have already established good rapport with the patient. Conversely, when a long-time patient presents in labour, the teacher may be reluctant to relinquish care to a learner, regardless of their competence. Thus, it is important to be aware of how a teacher's relationship with the patient may influence their willingness to "let go."

Involving Other Members of the Team in the Learning Process

There are many opportunities for the other members of the perinatal care team to become involved as teachers. Each group of practitioners has their unique body of knowledge and approach to patient care, which can benefit the undifferentiated learner in labour and delivery. Their expertise must be acknowledged as valuable, and their teaching efforts should be rewarded rather than seen as extra work. This is challenging from the individual teacher's point of view. However, the program might consider ways of showing appreciation to colleagues in other disciplines who are valuable teachers. Letters of appreciation, food baskets, or even special awards for teaching could be considered.

Labour and delivery nurses have much to offer learners in other professions, due to the fact that they have extensive expertise in labour management. Learners should be encouraged to take their cues from experienced nurses in terms of what is "normal" and what is concerning. Some situations where nurses can help with the teaching process include:

- Verifying vaginal exam findings
- Reviewing electronic fetal heart monitoring records
- Demonstrating supportive care in labour

- Managing the second stage (different positions, how to coach pushing, how to involve the partner)
- Immediate care of the newborn (supporting newborn transition, resuscitation if needed, early breastfeeding support)

Obstetricians are also valuable members of the teaching team. They may be primary teachers or may teach in a consultant role. Learners should present requests for consultation to the obstetrician (with the support of their supervising teacher) using an organized framework for communication between members of the healthcare team, such as the "SBAR" (situation, background, assessment, and recommendations) format (Shahid & Thomas, 2018), to demonstrate that the learner understands the reasons for the consult and the anticipated response from the specialist. Hearing the learner present the case allows the teacher to reflect on the learner's comprehension of the situation. It also encourages the learner's involvement in the further management of the case.

Anaesthetists have a valuable role in teaching learners about medical strategies for pain relief in labour, as well as resuscitation of unstable patients. The primary teacher should identify these learning opportunities, connect the learner with the anaesthetist, and debrief about the experience afterward.

Pediatricians and respiratory therapists (RTs) have expertise in neonatal resuscitation and assessment of the at-risk newborn. It is very useful for learners to work with these members of the healthcare team during both routine and emergency care. This might occur in an ad hoc way when there is downtime in L and D, when one of their patients requires these specialized services, or on a scheduled basis (e.g., by scheduling the learners to work one or two shifts with RTs).

Midwives have expertise in physiologic birth as well as out-of-hospital birth. It can be useful for learners in different professions to shadow and participate in midwife-attended births to learn strategies to facilitate normal birth as well as to understand the clinical scope and context of midwifery care. Similarly, it may be possible for other teachers to participate in the education of midwifery learners on the labour and delivery floor.

RETURN TO BACKSTAGE (AFTER THE BIRTH)

Debriefing Every Birth

Debriefing With the Team. Ideally, the core team members and birthing family should be involved in a debriefing after the birth.

Debriefing is an interactive conversation to reflect on performance, involving everyone who was at the birth. It acknowledges the value of staff input, reflection, and analysis of teamwork (Cheng et al., 2014). This allows the healthcare team to address any questions that the birthing family may have about the birth. Answering these questions with the learner present can be a learning experience for them in terms of the rationale for the management of the birth and the communication with the family.

Subsequently, the healthcare team members can debrief about the event, asking themselves, "What went well?" and "What do we think that we could have done better?" This is an opportunity to discuss possibilities for improvement—including "near misses"—for the benefit of the team, the learner, and future patients.

Debriefing With the Learner. There should be a debriefing between the teacher and learner, wherein the learner is provided with an opportunity to ask questions and reflect on what they learned. The teacher can summarize what they felt were the key learning points and provide additional feedback to what was already provided "in the moment." It is particularly important to debrief with the learner if there were high-stakes events or if the learner appeared overwhelmed by the situation or ensuing questions.

To clarify and distinguish the terminology that is often used in the context of debriefing, here are some helpful definitions:

- **Feedback** is an educational tool that supports the learner's growth. All teachers must be adept at feedback, which is most effective when applied within a trusting educational alliance in a non-judgmental, objective manner, close to the time of the event. In this context, we are referring to "formative" feedback. (See Chapter 10.)

  Example:

  "That delivery went really well because you supported the perineum well and there was no tear. Here is a little feedback for the next delivery: next

time, I would like to see you wait until the second contraction to deliver the shoulders. That way, the head has a chance to restitute, and you actually have a lower chance of getting a shoulder dystocia."

- **Coaching** is an educational philosophy that supports the learner's development in the following domains: knowledge and skills, professional trajectory, and personal growth. All of these aspects of learner growth are important and should be done intentionally by the teacher. Coaching can occur in the moment or over time, where the longitudinal relationship between learner and mentor allows the learner to reflect on their performance and develop new professional and personal objectives (Atkinson et al., 2021).

Example:

"Let's take advantage of this quiet moment on our call shift to talk about your future plans. You mentioned that you were interested in incorporating perinatal care into your future practice. What do you think you will need to accomplish this? How can I help you to achieve your goals?"

- **Learning conversations** are scheduled meetings to discuss medical questions, selected topics, or professional performance. They may include feedback and/or debriefing. However, they differ from immediate or impromptu feedback or debriefing in that they are deliberately planned and are primarily an opportunity for the learner to demonstrate self-directed learning and set their own learning goals (Welink et al., 2020).

Example:

"Thank you for meeting with me today to discuss your progress on the perinatal care rotation. Last time, you expressed that you were still feeling uncomfortable with perineal repair. Tell me how you have been practising this since we last met."

Special Considerations

ONE PATIENT BECOMES TWO

This chapter has focused on teaching during the labour and birth. However, unique to the experience of the comprehensive healthcare provider is the fact that after every successful birth there is a second patient to care for. Many learners are not aware of this expectation. The teaching tips described above can be transferred to the care of the newborn. Specific strategies for teaching breastfeeding, management of "the golden hour," and so forth, are provided in Chapter 5. However, immediate newborn care—patient-centred birth, delayed cord clamping, the importance of skin-to-skin contact, the complete newborn examination, the management of the newborn who requires resuscitation—is an area that should be role-modelled by the comprehensive practitioner and involve the learner.

Example:

You have just delivered a baby with a learner. The repair is complete, the mother is in a dry, clean bed, and the baby appears stable on her chest. The learner is writing the postpartum orders and is anxious to get on to other activities. You remind them that they have not examined the baby yet and they now have responsibility for two patients. The learner goes to take the baby over to the warmer for the examination and weight when you stop them, saying: "I understand that you are keen to weigh and examine the baby. However, this first hour of skin-to-skin is very important for mother-infant bonding and the initiation of breastfeeding. Let us arrange to meet back in about an hour if the activity on labour and delivery permits. We can review the normal newborn exam—and, in particular, how to conduct it on the mother. Weighing the baby can wait."

THE MALE LEARNER

Perinatal care is a core part of medical training in Canada and is required for all learners, regardless of gender. However, what individual learners actually experience in perinatal care may differ greatly based on their gender (Zahid,

2015). This is often because female patients may decline the participation of male learners for multiple reasons:

- Religious reasons
- Previous sexual trauma
- Belief that female care providers might understand them better
- Partner preference

Regardless of the reason, when a male learner is declined participation in the healthcare team, there is a broad ripple effect, and there are implications for the teacher, the learner, the patient, and the profession.

Introducing the concept of learners (and in particular, male learners) in perinatal care starts in the office (see Chapter 1). Patients should be introduced to the role of learners in the healthcare team and the importance of the patient in the educational process. There is increased male learner acceptance into sensitive patient encounters when educational messages about training are delivered by a credible source (Buck & Littleton, 2016).

THE LEARNER WITH "BAD HANDS"

Unlike surgical trainees, who are often screened for manual dexterity, learners in a generalist program arrive with various abilities. It is frustrating for the teacher and the learner when it is evident that the learner is not progressing in the expected manner when it comes to manual skills—particularly suturing. Some suggestions for this situation include . . .

- Backstage: Direct the learner to practise away from the patient. This reduces stress for the learner and permits repetition to the point of "muscle memory." Many models exist for knot-tying and suturing—from extremely basic to those that use a pig's anus (which can be obtained from a butcher shop) to simulate the perineum. There are also many YouTube videos to assist with knot-tying and perineal repair. The teacher should encourage the learner to strive for proficiency in one-handed knots and basic suturing skills before applying them to a patient. For more on simulation, see Chapter 4.
- Onstage: Give the learner clear direction regarding basic manipulation of instruments. Learners have likely not been taught how to mount a

needle onto a needle driver, safeguard themselves and others with pro-tected hand-offs, safely dispose of sharps, and so on.

MANAGEMENT OF OBSTETRIC EMERGENCIES

Obstetric and neonatal emergencies can be catastrophic for the birthing person and baby. In addition, there can be significant secondary trauma for care providers and learners who are involved in an emergency situation, particularly if the outcome is not favourable. In all settings, perinatal care providers are expected to stay current in the interprofessional management of obstetrical and neonatal emergencies. Where possible, learners should be involved in these programs, which might be individual (such as online courses), hospital-based drills (such as those developed by MORE[OB] or PROMPT (Practical Obstetric Multi-Professional Training)), or accredited national programs such as ALARM (Advances in Labour and Risk Management) or ALSO (Advanced Life Support in Obstetrics).

It is very important to support learners who have been involved in obstetrical emergencies or perinatal loss. Teachers should try to keep them involved in the ongoing care of the family after the event and invite learners to participate in formal case reviews. In addition, teachers should check in with the learner frequently to offer supportive strategies to cope with what may be their first experience with an adverse medical outcome.

OPPORTUNITIES FOR MENTORSHIP, CAREER COUNSELLING

As stated at the opening of this chapter, there are few teaching or learning experiences that are as intense as working one-on-one in labour and delivery for a 24-hour shift. There are almost always periods of downtime that can be used for various teaching opportunities. This chapter has already addressed using these times for problem-based learning, learning conversations, and so forth. However, the opportunity to use these times for mentorship and career counselling is often overlooked. Learners appreciate the opportunity to discuss their professional goals with a trusted teacher and appreciate when their teachers show interest in their personal and professional development.

REFERENCES

Atkinson, A., Watling, C.J., & Brand, P.L.P. (2021). Feedback and coaching. European Journal of Pediatrics, 181(2), 1-6. doi.org/10.1007/s00431-021-04118-8.

Biringer, A., Forte, M., Tobin, A., Shaw, E., & Tannenbaum, D. (2018). What influences success in family medicine maternity care education programs? Qualitative exploration. Canadian Family Physician, 64(5), e242-e248.

Buchmann, E., & Libhaber, E. (2008). Interobserver agreement in intrapartum estimation of fetal head station. International Journal of Gynecology & Obstetrics, 101(3), 285–289.

Buck, K., Littleton, H. (2016). Impact of educational messages on patient acceptance of male medical students in OB-Gyn encounters. Journal of Psychosomatic Obstetrics and Gynecology, 37(3), 84-90.

Carty, M., O'Riordan, N., Ivers, M., & Higgins, M.F. (2020). Patient perspectives of bedside teaching in an obstetrics, Gynaecology and neonatology hospital. BioMed Central Medical Education, 20, 111. https://doi.org/10.1186/s12909-020-02016-5

Cheng, A., Eppich, W., Grant, V., Sherbino, J., Zendejas, B., & Cook, D. (2014). Debriefing for technology-enhanced simulation: A systematic review. Medical Education, 48, 657-666.

Gingerich, A., Daniels, V., Farrell, L., Olsen, S.R., Kennedy, T., & Hatala, R. (2018). Beyond hands-on and hands-off: supervisory approaches and entrustment on the inpatient ward. Medical Education, 52(10), 1028-1040. doi: 10.1111/medu.13621.

Gluck, O., Mizrachi, Y., Ganer Herman, H., Bar, J., Kovo, M., & Weiner, E. (2020). The correlation between the number of vaginal examinations during active labour and febrile morbidity, a retrospective cohort study. Biomed Central Pregnancy Childbirth, 20, 246. https://doi.org/10.1186/s12884-020-02925-9

Güneş, G., & Karaçam, Z. (2017). The feeling of discomfort during vaginal examination, history of abuse and sexual abuse and post-traumatic stress disorder in women. Journal of Clinical Nursing, 26(15-16), 2362-2371. doi: 10.1111/jocn.13574.

Hernandez, J.E., Vasan, N., Huff, S., & Melovitz-Vasan, C. (2020). Learning styles/preferences among medical students: Kinesthetic learner's multimodal approach to learning anatomy. Medical Science Education, 30, 1633–1638. https://doi.org/10.1007/s40670-020-01049-1

Lajoie, S.P., & Gube, M. (2018). Adaptive expertise in medical education: accelerating learning trajectories by fostering self-regulated learning. Medical Teacher, 40, 809-812. https://doi.org/10.1080/0142159X.2018.1485886

Masters, P. (2020). What doctors can (and should) learn from patients. KevinMD.com, Jan 5, 2020.

Shahid, S., & Thomas, S. (2018). Situation, background, assessment, recommendation (SBAR) communication tool for handoff in health care – A narrative review. Safety and Health 4, 7. https://doi.org/10.1186/s40886-018-0073-1

Ten Cate, O., Hart, D., Ankel, F., Busari, J. Englander, R., Glasgow, N., Holmboe, E., Iobst, W., Lovell, E., Snell, L., Touchie, C., Van Melle, E., & Wycliffe-Jones, K. (2016). Entrustment decision making in clinical training. Academic Medicine, 91 (2), 191-198.doi: https://doi.org/10.1097/ACM.0000000000001044

Tobin, S., Biringer, A., Boutilier-Dean, M., Carroll, J., Medves, J., Oandasan, I., & Van Wagner, V. (2006). A Qualitative exploration of learners' experiences in maternity care education. The Babies Can't Wait Project. Technical Report #2. Toronto, ON: Ontario College of Family Physicians.

Welink, L., de Groot, E., Bartelink, M-L., Van Roy, K., Damoiseaux, R., & Pype, P. (2020). Learning conversations with trainees: An undervalued but useful EBM learning opportunity for clinical supervisors. Teaching and Learning in Medicine, 33 (4), 382-389. doi: 10.1080/10401334.2020.1854766

Whitman, N., & Magill, M. (2000). The teaching moment. In Paulman, P., Susman, J., & Abboud, C. (Eds), Precepting medical students in the office. Baltimore: The Johns Hopkins University Press.

Zahid, A. (2015.) Gender bias in O and G training: Does it matter? Poster presentation. 24th Asian and Oceanic Congress and Gynaecology. https://www.researchgate.net/publication/291832514_Gender_Bias_in_OG_Training_Does_it_matter

Chapter 4

SIMULATION-BASED LEARNING

Vicki Van Wagner, Rory Windrim

Dr. Janice McKeown is a new clinical teacher on call at the hospital and is working with a learner who tells her that they do not feel confident with internal exams and that they are nervous about where to put their hands when the cord is around the neck during birth. Dr. McKeown wants to find ways to demonstrate and practise with the learner. A midwifery colleague who is sitting beside her at the nursing station while they document over-hears the conversation and suggests that Janice and the learner could share the midwifery simulation models to practise assessing dilation, effacement, and station and fetal position using old socks and a doll. The midwife also shows Janice some websites with instructions for making a pelvic model from cardboard and explains how to make an umbilical cord from yarn to practise handling a nuchal cord.

Simulation has been used for centuries all over the world to teach perinatal care skills in a safe manner (Carty, 2010), providing the opportunity for what 17th-century obstetrician Sir Richard Manningham called "forming your hands for practice" (Gardner & Raemer, 2008). In recent years, there has been an expansion of the role of simulation beyond its facilitation of the acquisition of manual skills. It is becoming a cornerstone tool in quality improvement, risk management, and patient safety programs. In the latter situation, simulation is designed to improve both individual and team clinical performances while reducing the risk of medical and communication errors. In this chapter, we will briefly introduce the main educational concepts of simulation-based learning. We will review the two main educational uses of simulation: practical skill acquisition with both low- and high-fidelity equipment and subsequent incorporation of these strategies into team-based roleplaying simulations with a focus on immersive and experiential team learning.

What is the evidence to support simulation-based learning?

- Simulation results in the more effective transfer of knowledge from expert to novice and works to "shorten the learning curve" (McLaughlin et al., 2008; Johannsson et al., 2005; Fransen et al., 2020)
- The use of simulation in the education of medical, midwifery, and nursing learners improves learner satisfaction, confidence, skills, decision-making, and test scores (Cant, 2010; Merien et al., 2010)
- Medical and midwifery learners display more competence and confidence and participate more actively in labour and delivery if they receive simulation training in normal birth (Andrighetti, 2012)
- Clinical evidence for improved care and outcomes is strong for emergency skills such as management of shoulder dystocia, postpartum hemorrhage, assisted vaginal birth, and breech birth for those who have engaged in simulation-based learning (Lendahls & Oscarsson, 2017)

What are the benefits of simulation-based learning?

- Repetitive practice of manoeuvres or procedures prior to their use in a clinical situation
- The ability for the teacher to give feedback in a safe space for everyone involved
- The learner's exposure to a range of difficulties for the procedure
- The learner's exposure to uncommon events
- The ability for teachers to assess their learners
- The absence of risks to patients (Okuda et al., 2009; Merien et al., 2010; Johannsson, 2005; Ennen & Satin, 2010; Satin, 2018).

Example:

It is 3 a.m. and you decide that a fetal scalp electrode (FSE) is required because the fetal heart tracing is atypical and there are technical issues with identifying it with the abdominal transducer. You ask the learner about their experience with the application of an FSE. After a brief discussion about the challenges they have encountered, the learner is permitted to use the FSE (which you keep on the labour floor in the "teachers' toolbox") to practise while you provide immediate feedback. When the first application goes well, you increase the station of the simulated fetal head and apply lubricant to the learner's gloves to raise the level of difficulty. After this, the learner feels ready to apply the electrode in the clinical situation.

The opportunity to "make mistakes without any risk to the patient, themselves, or other team members" (Johannsson, 2005) is a major benefit of simulated practice for learners (Ennen & Satin, 2010). Learners often find it easier to accept feedback and correct errors in a lower-stress simulation environment rather than in the midst of clinical care. Teachers can find it easier to follow up a learner's misstep by walking through a simulation, allowing the learner to demonstrate that the teacher's feedback has been understood and integrated. Simulation can also provide the opportunity to learn from mistakes. It can complement the tips and clinical stories passed on by an experienced practitioner.

What are the challenges in simulation-based learning?

- The expense of equipment and its maintenance and storage
- The need for time and space for learners and teachers to work together
- The requirement for learner "buy-in" and faculty commitment
- The limitations to replication of complex clinical situations
- The limitations to accurate learner assessment (Draycott et al, 2015, Fox-Young et al, 2012).

It is important to contextualize simulation for learners and to be clear about its purpose(s). Simulations can act as preparation for hands-on tasks, remediation for when skills need development, opportunities to practise for uncommon events that cannot be learned in clinical settings alone, or methods of evaluation.

More evidence is emerging about the level of fidelity needed for particular skills and the limits of what can be learned (Ennen & Satin, 2010; Merien et al., 2010; Massouth et al., 2019; Garvey & Dempsey, 2020). It helps when teachers acknowledge the limitations. Practising perineal repair on a foam model helps learners acquire the techniques and feel comfortable with the steps of the procedure, but it is not a substitute for learning how to assess a real tear. There are limits to the value of using simulation for assessment. Some learners may be able to perform well in simulations but struggle in clinical situations. The reverse can also be true. Simulation can enhance the learning process as well as support respectful, high-quality, person-centred care. However, it should always be used as an adjunct to—not a substitute for—clinical experience (Cooper et al., 2012).

How should teachers choose between low- and high-fidelity simulations?

There is good evidence for both low- and high-fidelity mannequins, but there are strengths and limitations of both (Ennen & Satin, 2010; Merien et al., 2010; Finan et al., 2019; Massouth et al., 2019). Once a decision has been made that simulation would be an appropriate teaching technique, the most commonly used method is simple simulation (Berg et al., 2015). The materials and techniques are available to all teachers, whereas the high-fidelity mannequins are less accessible. The following sections describe many techniques to make simple simulation models. As some hospitals have high-fidelity simulation labs, this will be covered in a following segment.

Simple Simulation

The process of constructing simple simulation models is central to their value. The act of making the model is a significant part of learner education, by encouraging them to apply their knowledge of anatomy and the procedure itself. Making a model can increase retention of information and tactile skill. The teacher can consider constructing a model with the learner as part of the practice session or have the learner make the model, practise at home, and debrief via photos or videos. Models should be as simple as possible, depending on the skill, the level of the learner, and the context in which they are used. The goal is to deepen learning and competence, not to create a perfect model. Handmade simulations used in combination with commercial pelvic models or obstetric mannequins can make the simulation more realistic, but simple pelvic models made of cardboard can be effective and more accessible in community settings. Simple simulations may help to demystify skills and procedures and do not require the training required for many of the high-fidelity models. See Fig. 1, below, for the required equipment to construct simple simulations.

Skill	Equipment
Assessment of cervical dilation and effacement	Jar lids, doll and socks, needle and thread, plastic wrap, Play-Doh©, pelvic model if desired
Determining presentation and position	Plastic lids or a grapefruit, pelvic model if desired
Stretch and sweep	Doll and socks, plastic wrap, pelvic model if desired
Pushing back an anterior lip	Doll and socks, plastic wrap, pelvic model if desired
Assessment and rupture of membranes	Doll and socks, balloons, plastic wrap, pelvic model if desired
Application of fetal scalp electrode (FSE)	Doll and socks, FSE, pelvic model if desired
Cervical ripening with balloon catheter and other methods	Plastic bottle, sponge, balloon catheter, speculum, pelvic model, and doll if desired
Urinary catheterization	Kitchen sponge and balloon, urinary catheter, pelvic model if desired
Conduct of vaginal birth (including nuchal cord or emergency management)	Doll and pelvic model, birth instruments
Cord blood collection	Yarn cord, urinary catheter, syringe, needles
Episiotomy	Doll, sock, scissors, pelvic model if desired
Perineal repair	Foam block, meat or cloth model and suturing equipment

FIGURE 1. EQUIPMENT REQUIRED TO CONSTRUCT SIMPLE SIMULATIONS FOR SKILLS TEACHING.

The following is a description of specific clinical skills that can be taught using simple simulation.

THE INTERNAL EXAMINATION

Internal examinations are intimidating for the learner and—given their intimate nature—can be uncomfortable for the labouring person. Thus, internal examination is a skill ideally suited to learning by simulation. It is difficult for learners to know what to feel for when they first begin conducting internal exams in labour. Simulation can make the invisible *visible*, and benefits both tactile and visual learners.

Assessment of Cervical Dilation and Effacement

Use household objects such as jar lids to learn dilation. Ask learners to find different sized lids from 1 to 10 centimetres and label them. For beginners, the labels visible on the front help create a pattern of recognition from learners' fingers to their brains, acting as self-assessment tools (see Fig. 2).

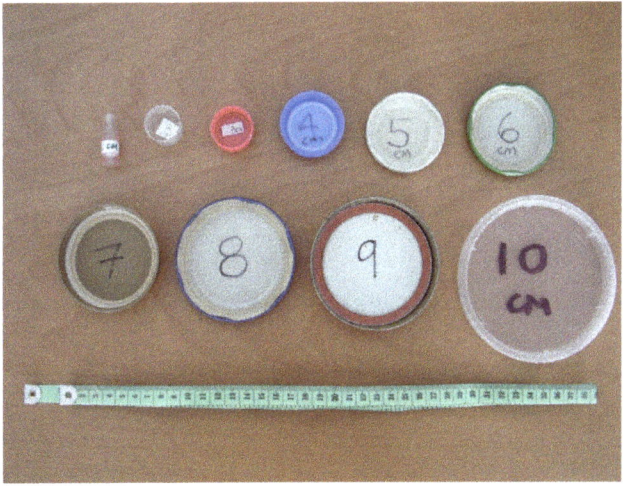

FIGURE 2: JAR LIDS FOR LEARNING DILATION.

Socks and dolls are easy to use to create cervical models to practise assessing both cervical effacement and dilation. To do so, you should . . .

1. Cut old socks into tubes pulled over a doll's head
2. Make different sized openings in the toe of the sock or by pulling the cuff to different diameters around the doll's head, creating different dilations

3. Use socks of various thicknesses to create different effacements
4. Use the doll and sock models in combination with a commercial pelvic model or obstetric mannequin to make the simulation more realistic. Figure 3 shows a cloth pelvis and a posterior sock cervix.

The following illustrations demonstrate the construction of this model.

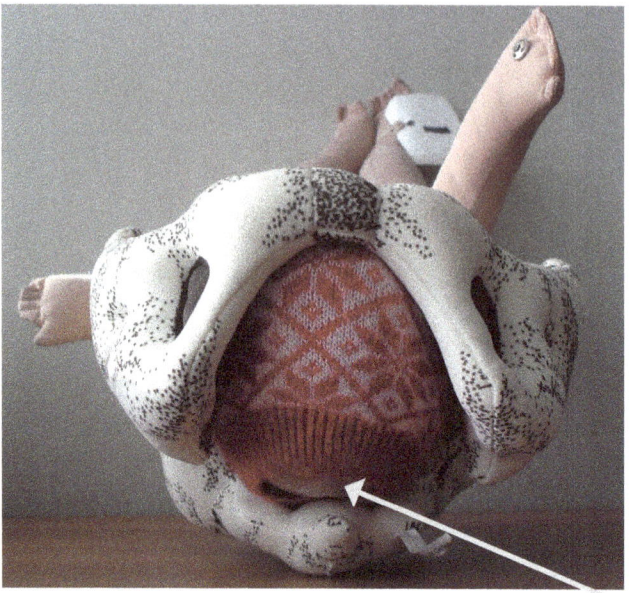

FIGURE 3: SOCK CERVIX, DOLL, AND PELVIS.   Cervical os

If a commercial pelvic model or mannequin is not available, a simple cardboard box pelvis can be a good substitute. If learners are interested, they can make a more anatomically correct cardboard pelvis. Instructions for how to make an anatomically correct cardboard pelvis can be found online (Lai, 2004).

Teachers can use these models to show common challenges and complications discovered on internal exam. For example, a very effaced cervix can be mistaken for bulging membranes. Making a "layered cervix" by sewing a thicker sock over a thinner sock demonstrates how practitioners can mistakenly assess dilation as 6 centimetres because they have not clearly identified the two-centimetre os (Fig. 4).

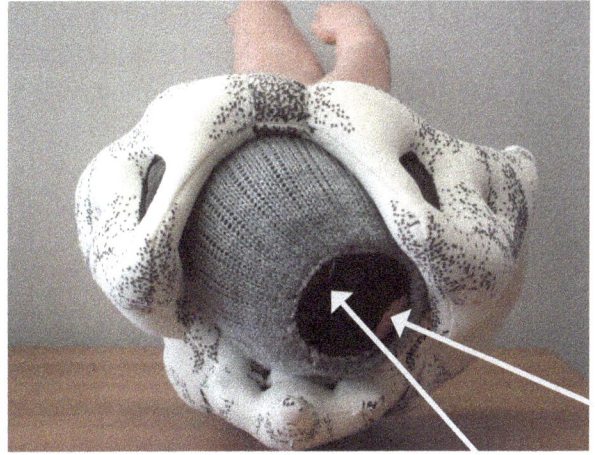

FIGURE 4: LAYERED CERVIX.   Layer of cervix

Cervical os

Identifying Cord Prolapse or Vasa Previa

The identification of these rare but critical findings can be practised using doll, sock, pelvis or mannequin, and a yarn cord for cord prolapse (Fig. 5) or a urinary catheter and plastic wrap for vasa previa. You can make an inexpensive umbilical cord using different colours of yarn. Instructions for making a yarn cord can be found online (Dziegnel, 2016).

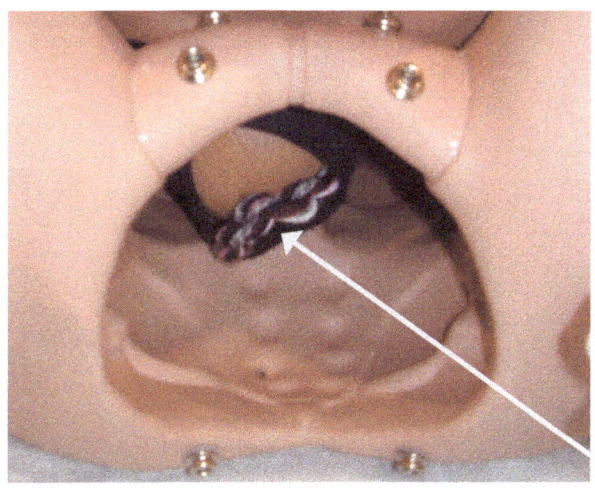

Yarn cord

FIGURE 5: YARN USED TO MODEL CORD PROLAPSE

Determining Presentation and Position

Use dolls and pelvic models so that the learner can identify the landmarks for various presentations. Commercial models have limitations, as they do not demonstrate the overlap of bones with moulding, though they help with understanding anatomy (Fig. 6). For non-vertex presentations, use a doll or baby mannequin, having learners palpate the triangle of the mouth and malar bones in a face presentation (Fig. 7) and the straight line of the ischial tuberosities and the anus in a breech (Fig. 8).

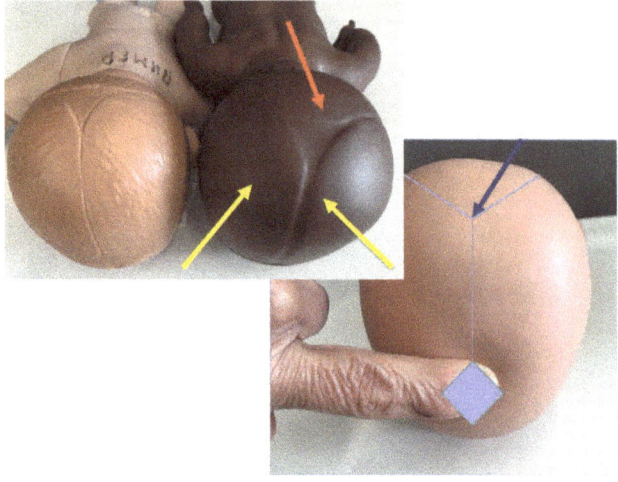

FIGURE 6: USING COMMERCIAL DOLLS TO LEARN FETAL LANDMARKS.

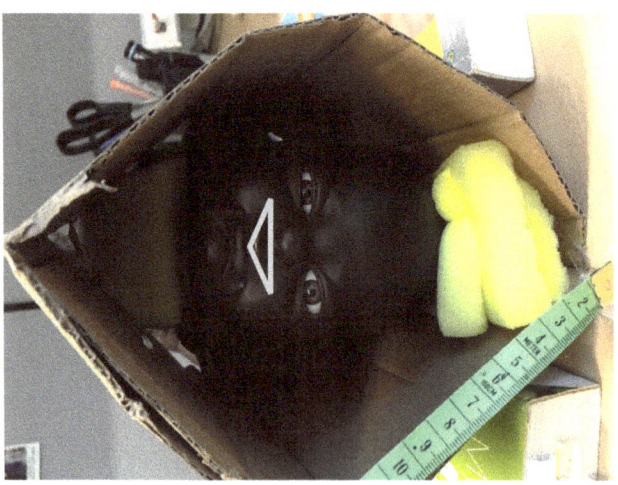

FIGURE 7: USING A DOLL AND CARDBOARD PELVIS TO IDENTIFY FACE PRESENTATION.

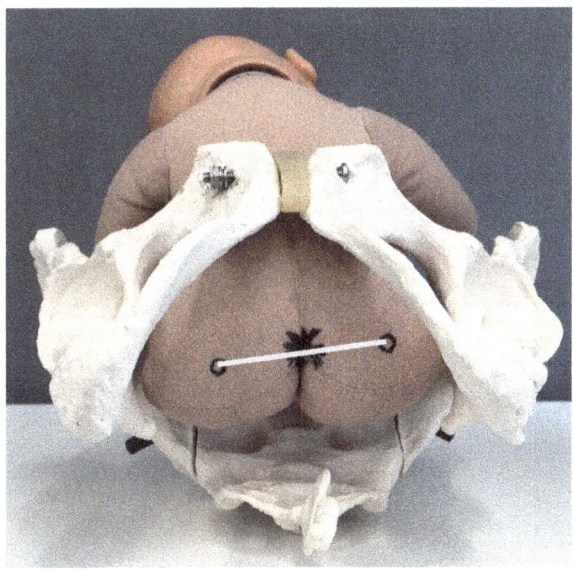

FIGURE 8: IDENTIFYING BREECH PRESENTATION.

To enhance learning about how to determine position in vertex presentation, learners can create and label a model of fetal skull landmarks using plastic lids (Fig. 9) for occiput anterior (OA) and occiput posterior (OP). To make a more anatomically correct version that has the round shape of a head, use a ball or the peel of a grapefruit. While making this model, learners should apply knowledge from texts about how the fetal skull bones overlap in occipital anterior and occipital posterior positions. Using this model, they can feel the overlap of the bones as they would during an intrapartum internal exam.

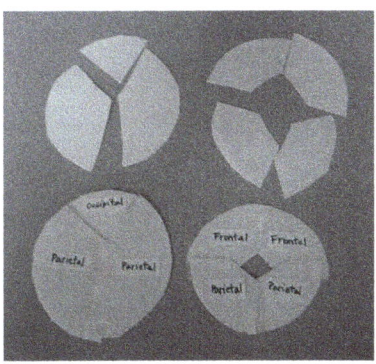

FIGURE 9: PLASTIC LID MODEL OF FETAL SKULL LANDMARKS.

Sweeping Membranes

Make cervical models for sweeping membranes by creating a long uneffaced cervix with a sock held together with elastics of varying tightness. Cover a doll's head with a layer of plastic wrap to mimic the feel of intact membranes and place the sock cervix over the plastic wrap (Fig. 10). Pelvic or vaginal models can add realism.

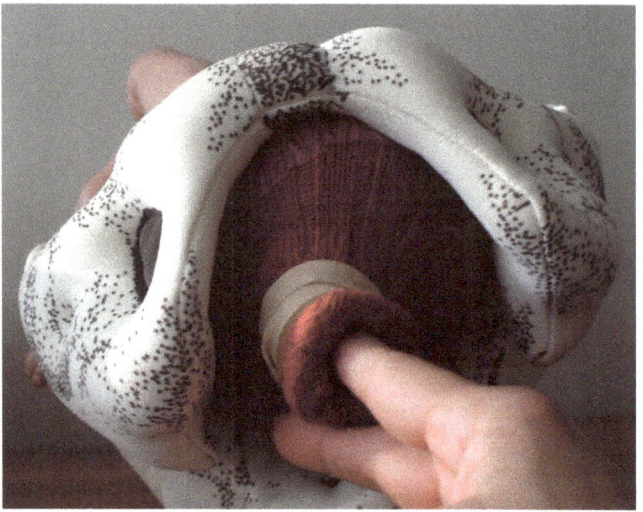

FIGURE 10: SOCK MODEL FOR STRETCH AND SWEEP.

Pushing Back an Anterior Lip

To make a model to practise "slipping a lip" over the occiput, wrap a thick, soft piece of sock in a long piece of plastic wrap. Fix it to the doll's head by using the rest of the plastic wrap (Fig. 11). Make sure you are able to push it back over the occiput. Place the doll in a pelvis or mannequin that is tight enough to mimic the feel of the anterior lip caught between the head and the pubic bone (Fig. 12). You can also use a sock to make a thin rim of cervix all around the vertex, which is often present with an anterior lip.

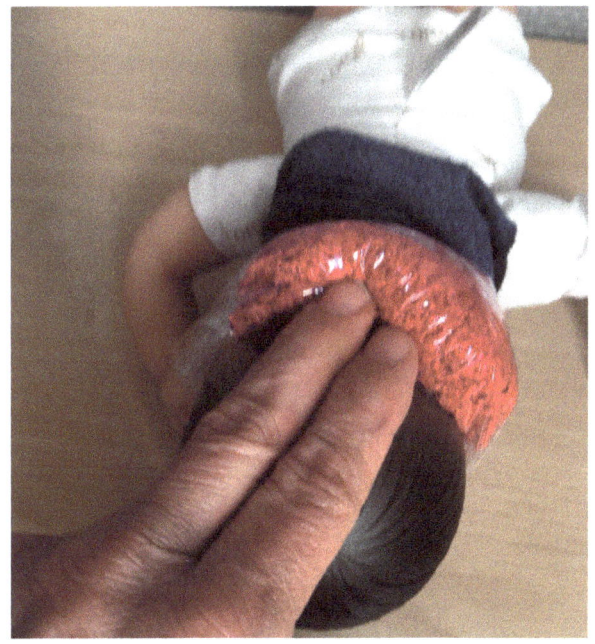

FIGURE 11: ANTERIOR LIP MODEL WITH SOCK AND PLASTIC WRAP.

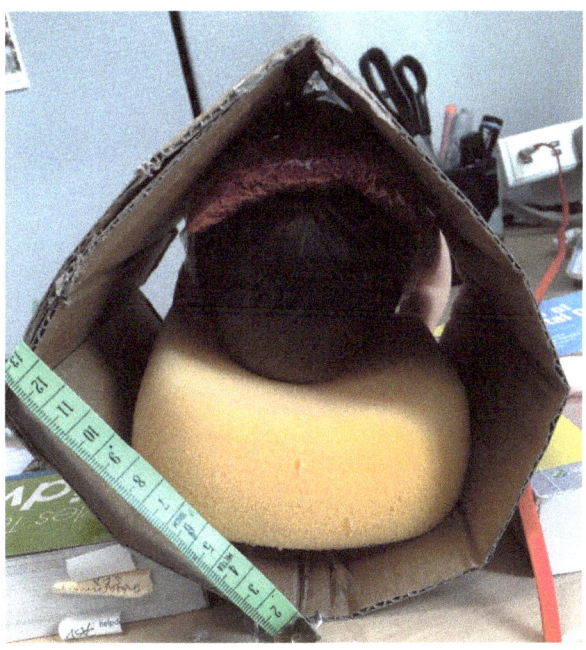

FIGURE 12: ANTERIOR LIP MODEL IN A CARDBOARD PELVIS.

Assessment and Artificial Rupture of Fetal Membranes (ARM)

Use this model with a sock cervix and/or with pelvis or mannequin. It provides an excellent setup to practise amniotomy or for use in a cord prolapse scenario.

1. Place a balloon on a doll's head and cover it with a layer of plastic wrap to simulate the two layers of fetal membranes
2. Pull the plastic wrap tightly over the doll's head using elastic bands or tape it around the doll's neck to secure the "membranes" (Fig. 13)

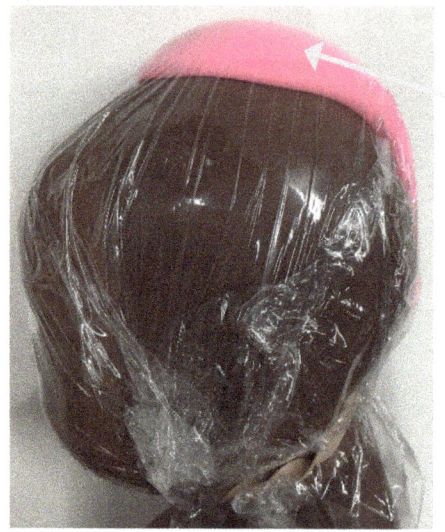

Balloon

FIGURE 13: USE OF BALLOON AND PLASTIC WRAP TO CREATE MEMBRANES.

3. Fill the balloon with more or less air or water to simulate degrees of bulging membranes
4. Place plastic wrap directly on the doll's head to simulate tight membranes that are difficult to assess and rupture (Fig. 14). Use lubricating gel to make the membranes feel slippery under gloved fingers. Use a pelvis or mannequin to increase the realism (Fig. 15).

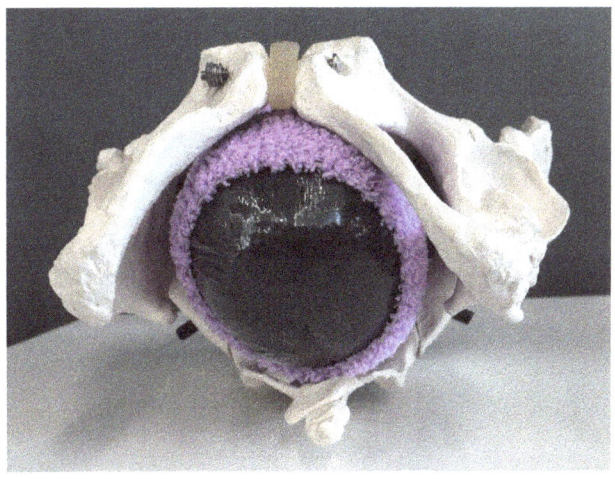

FIGURE 14: MODEL FOR RUPTURE OF TIGHT MEMBRANES.

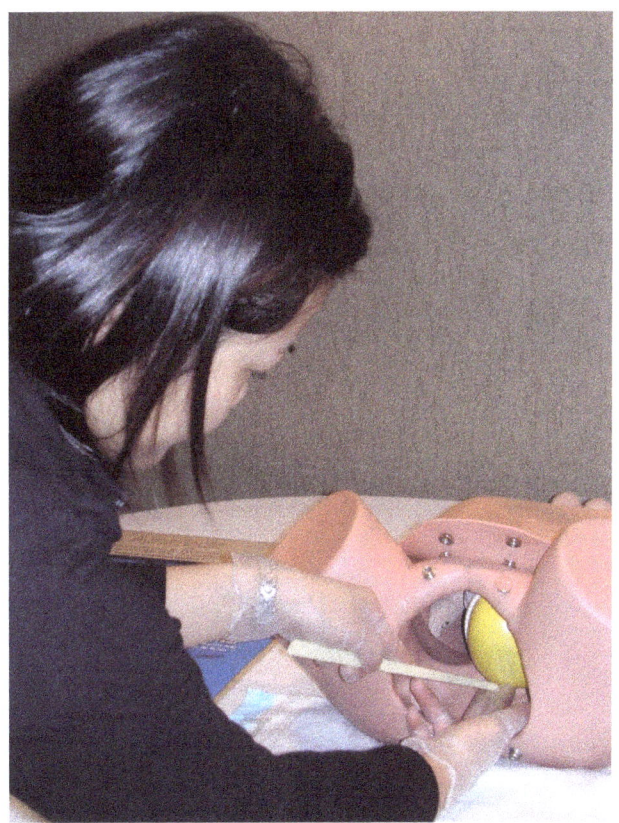

FIGURE 15: LEARNING ARM WITH A BALLOON MODEL.

Application of a Fetal Scalp Electrode

To teach how to apply and remove a fetal scalp electrode (FSE) . . .

1. Get a doll, a thick sock, and another sock of any kind
2. Put a thick sock over the doll's head—this is the layer used to insert the scalp electrode
3. Use another sock with a 6–7 centimetre opening over the thick sock—this sock is the cervical opening

Use this model in a pelvis or mannequin and with the plastic bottle vaginal model described below to make it more realistic.

With this model, the learner should prepare and apply the FSE. Using a commercial doll with an anatomical skull allows the student to include landmarking for placement of the FSE on the parietal bone rather than over a suture or fontanelle (Fig. 16).

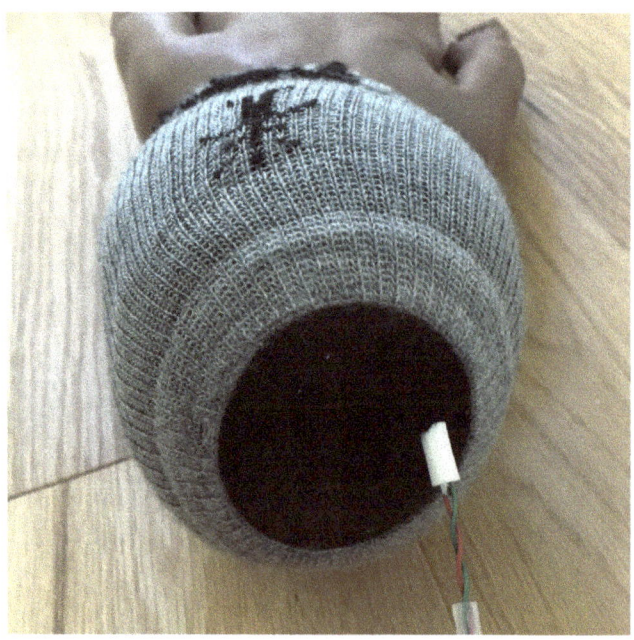

FIGURE 16: SOCK MODEL BEING USED FOR THE APPLICATION OF FSE.

Cervical Ripening

Use a plastic water bottle to make a vagina and a cervix and practise insertion of a balloon catheter, prostaglandin gel, or insert.

1. Cut the top and the bottom off the plastic water bottle. The plastic tube portion will become the vagina (Fig. 17).
2. Use the bottle opening for the cervix. Adding "the neck" of a balloon adds colour for visualization and gives it a smoother/slipperier surface.
3. Invert the top portion of the bottle and tape it at the top of the vaginal canal. Tilt it down to mimic the unripe cervix in a posterior position.
4. Cover the vaginal walls with foam so that you can use a speculum to visualize the cervix
5. Tape the model to a surface in order to stabilize it. Insert a speculum and balloon catheter. You can also use the model to apply prostaglandin gel or a prostaglandin insert (see Figs. 18 and 19).

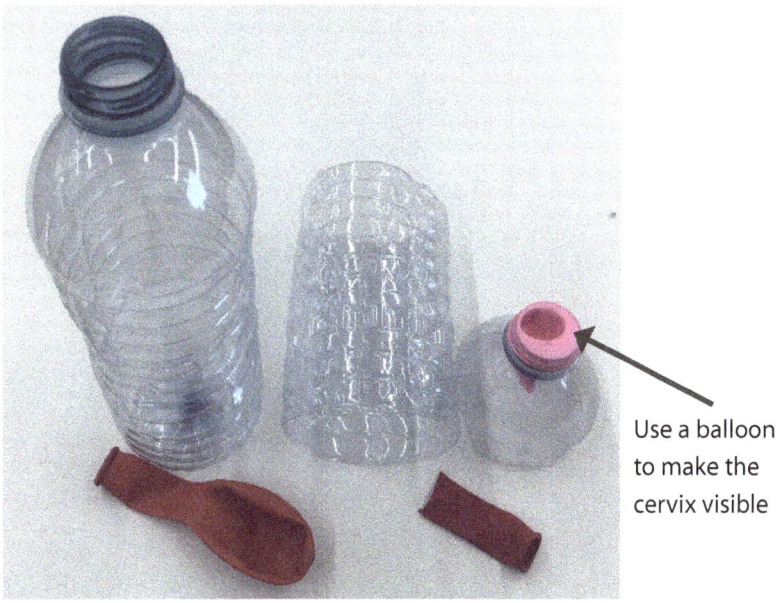

Use a balloon to make the cervix visible

FIGURE 17: PLASTIC BOTTLE AND BALLOON BEING USED TO MAKE A VAGINAL AND CERVIX.

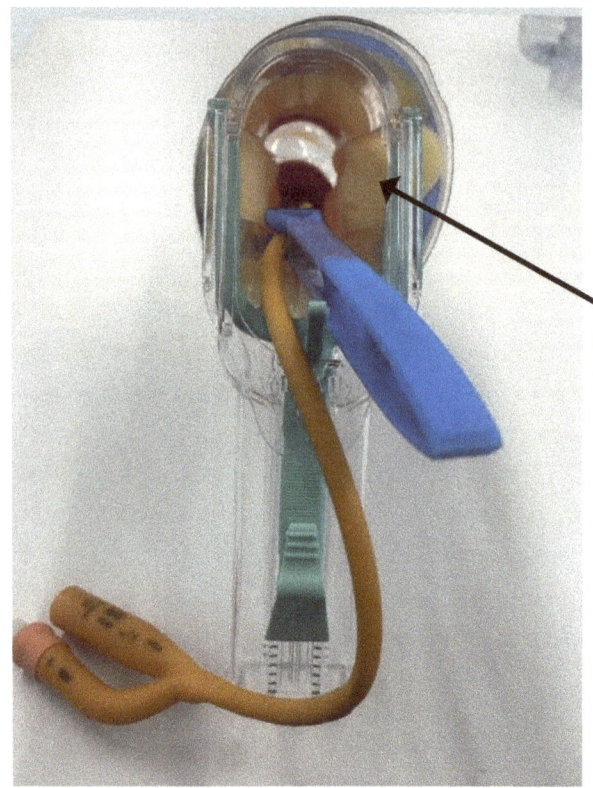

Use a sponge to line the bottle

FIGURE 18: INSERTION OF THE CATHETER.

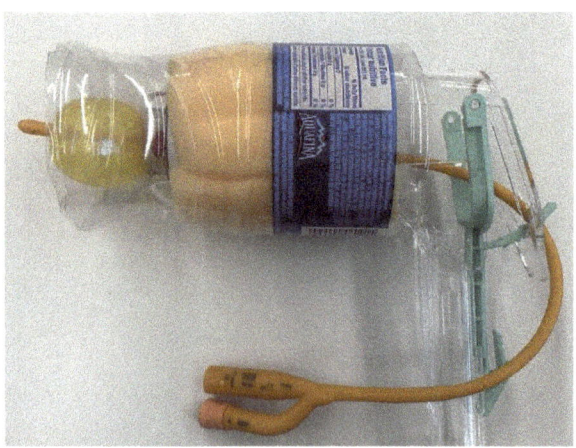

FIGURE 19: MODEL ONCE BALLOON IS BLOWN UP.

CONDUCT OF VAGINAL BIRTH

With a simple doll and pelvis or a commercial mannequin you can practise "catching" a baby with the learner. This can facilitate learning hand manoeuvres, practising how to communicate with the parents, and working together with other care providers. Some high-fidelity models mimic the perineum stretching more effectively than homemade or low-fidelity commercial models, but for most learners just roleplaying where to put their hands and what to say as the head descends and crowns helps them to feel more at ease in clinical settings.

There are tips to help effectively teach the conduct of vaginal birth using lower-fidelity commercial mannequins.

Most programs have these models, which include the plastic pelvis and baby. Consider the following when using these models:

- The plastic perineum is stiff and may inhibit teaching and learning. Use the perineum if teaching basic hand positions for birth but remove it when teaching breech or shoulder dystocia manoeuvres.
- The teacher has to move the doll through the pelvis as well as instruct or give feedback to the learner
- The instructor can roleplay the labouring person and use the pelvis or mannequin as "part of their body." The way the instructor and learners treat the mannequin can role-model respectful and person-centred care.
- The simulation can integrate more than procedural skills, including communication with the labouring person, communication with other care providers, and teamwork in emergencies

Management Of Nuchal Cord

To practise management of a nuchal cord, make a model with a doll, pelvis, and yarn cord (Fig. 20). You can use a cardboard or commercial pelvis or mannequin. Use this simple equipment with clamps and scissors to walk through the steps of looping the cord over the head, looping the cord over the shoulders, using the somersault manoeuvre (Fig. 21), or clamping and cutting a tight cord (Fig. 22).

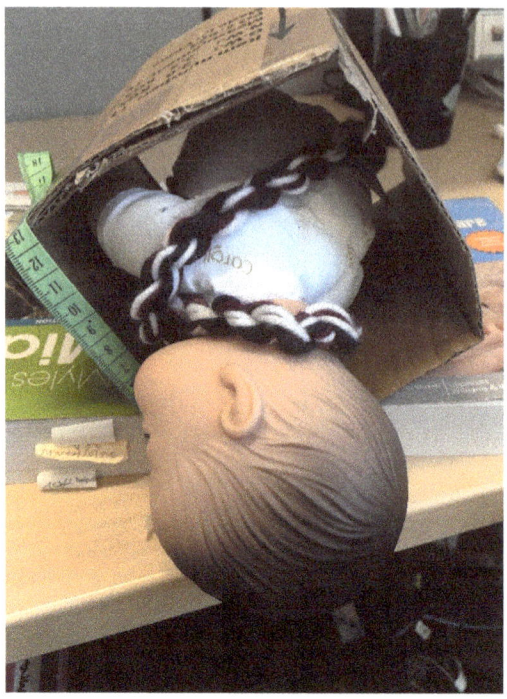

FIGURE 20: MODEL BEING USED TO PRACTISE MANAGEMENT OF NUCHAL CORD.

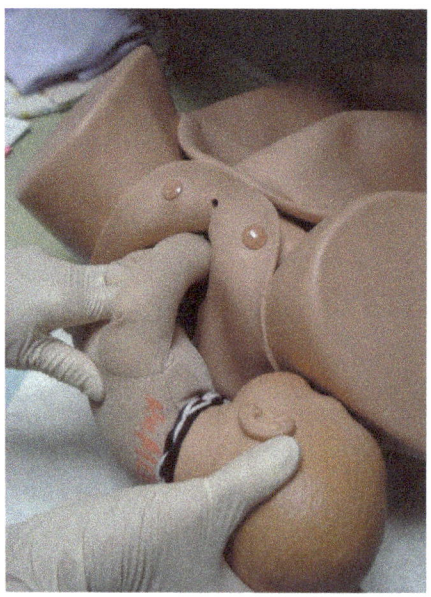

FIGURE 21: SOMERSAULT MANOEUVRE.

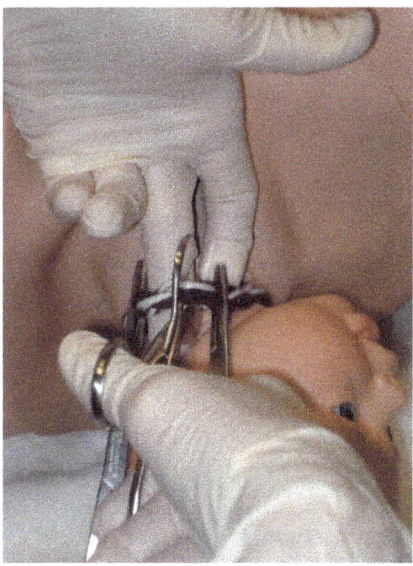

FIGURE 22: CLAMPING AND CUTTING A TIGHT CORD.

EPISIOTOMY

One model for teaching episiotomy uses a doll, a sock, and a pair of scissors—ideally in a pelvis or mannequin. In this scenario, the sock is the perineum (Fig. 23). Learners can demonstrate and practise the technique, allowing evaluation of this procedure. Roleplaying allows the teacher to assess how the learner explains the indications for the episiotomy and how they obtain informed consent.

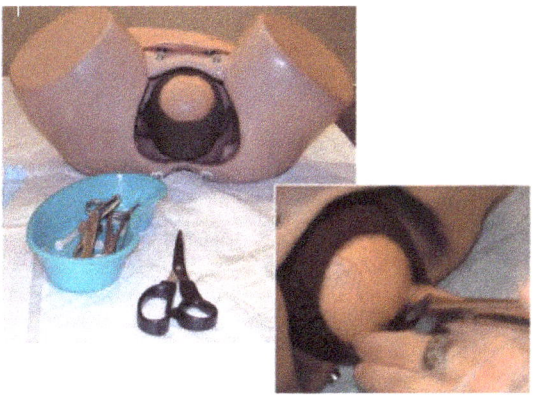

FIGURE 23: USING A SOCK MODEL TO PRACTISE EPISIOTOMY.

PERINEAL REPAIR

There are a variety of simple models for perineal repair, including with the use of foam blocks (Fig. 24), meat, or cloth models. Setups for simple simulations and commercial models for perineal repair are shown in many open access videos. Doing a "talk through" of these videos with a learner can provide a low-stress way to clarify understanding prior to simulated practice.

Suturing videos using simple simulation include:

- How to repair a 2nd degree perineal tear: a suturing workshop (Ting, 2020)
- Perineal Repair: Yellow sponge simulator 2nd degree tear (Laporte, 2012)

Suturing videos using commercial models include:

- Managing Obstetrical Trauma- Perineal suturing model (Blom, 2022)
- Perineal Repair (Hammond, 2014)

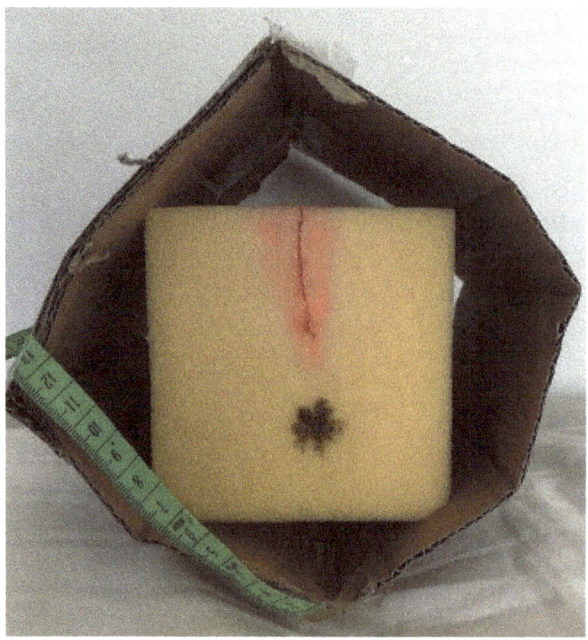

FIGURE 24: USING A SPONGE MODEL FOR SUTURING WITH A CARDBOARD BOX PELVIS.

CORD BLOOD COLLECTION

Use blue and red yarn and a phlebotomy kit to make a simulation for drawing cord blood. A urinary catheter filled with red fluid and woven into the yarn cord can make the simulation even more realistic (Fig. 25).

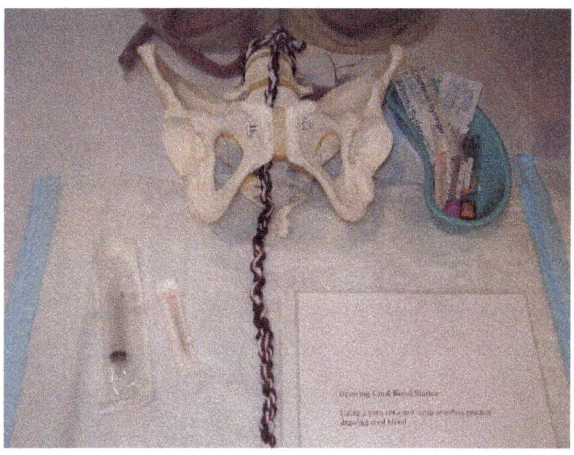

FIGURE 25: USING A YARN CORD TO PRACTISE CORD BLOOD COLLECTION.

CONCLUSION

In summary, the possibilities for simple simulations are endless and spark creativity for both learners and teachers as they use materials at hand. Using household objects to create simple models for clinical learning is, in our experience, popular with learners and highly ranked in program evaluations. The atmosphere of creativity and playfulness models resourcefulness, piques interest, and actively involves students in their learning.

High-Fidelity Simulation

High-fidelity birthing simulators are custom manufactured mannequins that enable highly realistic simulation of labour and delivery—both complicated and uncomplicated. There is a range of technological sophistication in the birth simulators available. This range of complexity and fidelity is matched by the costs involved in both purchasing and maintaining them (Costiuc, 2021).

At the simple end of this range are latex fetal and birthing models which, while highly realistic in appearance, are otherwise inert. Many birthing units can afford these simple mannequins, and they can be easily stored with zero maintenance requirements. These simulators, like the simple low-cost simulators detailed above, are commonly used for practising specific manoeuvres, both uncomplicated—as in normal birth—and complicated—such as in the case of shoulder dystocia (Costiuc, 2021).

At the complex end of this range are mechanized, technologically complex, full-body mannequins that are obstetric modifications of the well-established, sophisticated simulators employed in simulated CPR education. They can be pre-programmed and/or remotely controlled to move a fetal model through a simulated pelvis. These highly technical models are increasingly wireless and allow remotely controlled modulation of many aspects of the simulated birthing person/fetal anatomy and physiology. These mannequins are full size, can speak, and have cardiac and respiratory activity that are both visible and palpable, reactive pupils, movable limb joints, and more. All vital signs can be programmed to respond to interventions, such as administered medications. Obstetric functions include a dilating cervix, palpable uterine contractions with matched monitor patterns, and fetal heartrate monitor tracing. A motorized piston pushes the fetal mannequin through the birth canal at a pre-programmed or remotely controlled rate. Makeup, sometimes called *moulage* (e.g., fake blood), may be added to the mannequin in order to enhance the realism of the scenario. After delivery, newborn simulators with heartrate, respiratory rate, umbilical cord, and variable cyanosis are available, while postpartum hemorrhage (PPH) can be simulated with profuse "bleeding" through the mannequin's vagina and an uncontracted uterus.

These motorized, highly complex simulator mannequins provide very realistic experiences for teams that are evaluating their communications and interactions. The storage and deployment of these complex mannequins uses more labour, space, and capital. As such, their acquisition is often more appropriate for designated simulation areas or centres where the entire birthing or operating room environment can be simulated, and the mannequins form the central focus for practice for the entire healthcare team (Costiuc, 2010). Examples of high-fidelity mannequins include babies, Newborn Anne and SimNewB, or birthing patients, Noelle and Lucina, which can range in cost from approximately $3,000 to $88,000 CAD.

Roleplaying Team Simulations

While the mannequins described above are essential for practising specific procedures or manoeuvres, when the educational goal is to optimize team responses to an emergent or deteriorating clinical situation, an immersive simulation scenario might be most appropriate. In these scenarios, the maternal-fetal mannequin is employed as the central focus of a simulated obstetric event, either normal or complicated. These standardized scenarios can then be repetitively used for small group learning and evaluation.

Developing a Simulation

The following are important factors when it comes to developing a simulation.

1. *Structure:* The structure of the simulation should suit the purpose. Is it a quick debrief or a formal course or evaluation of a skill?

2. *Equipment:* Consider the equipment you have available in your setting. Generally, it is good to keep the equipment as simple as possible—being creative will help lower costs.

3. *Instructors:* Consider the number of instructors you need or have. For sessions focused on skills enhancement and practice, one instructor per model may work well, with the instructor integrating the role of the labouring person and the teacher (as described earlier in this chapter). For formal sessions that include strict time limits and evaluation, having two instructors at a station allows for more accurate assessment, as one instructor runs the scenario and moves the doll through the pelvis while the other observes the learner and uses an evaluation tool to assess performance.

4. *Scenarios:* Teachers may create scenarios on the spot for a quick session integrated into a clinic day or after a birth. Formal scenarios designed as part of a course or an evaluation process may support newer teachers. Scenarios can also aid with the integration of communication and interprofessional teamwork skills. Developing a perinatal simulation

scenario for experiential team learning is time- and effort-consuming, and involves detailed planning (Bambini, 2016; Harrington, 2021).

The steps involved are as follows:

- Choose the specific aspect(s) of the individual's/team's knowledge or function to be reviewed. For example, a PPH station could be designed to evaluate the clinical management and team communication.
- Develop an appropriate clinical story and provide specific roles and scripts for all relevant professions involved in the case.
- Decide the tools required for the scenario, including the physical environment (labour and delivery room versus triage area, etc.) and patient/family actors if appropriate, as well as the level of simulator fidelity needed, and any other equipment or supplies that may be necessary.
- Develop instructions for faculty, standardized patients, learners, and so on. These instructions will inform the three phases of the station: prebrief, scenario completion, and debrief.
- Conduct a practice run-through to identify potential timing or other problems.

The team can make their own scenario de novo or utilize one of the generic scenario templates that have been published. Alternatively, the team could choose to use their simulation resources within an established safe birth simulation program, such as ALARM (Advances in Labour and Risk Management) (Windrim et al., 2006), MORE[OB] (Managing Obstetric Risk Efficiently) (Reszel et al.. 2019), the Canadian Association of Midwives Emergency Skills Program (Canadian Association of Midwives, 2021), PROMPT (Practical Obstetric Multi-Professional Training) (Abdelrahman & Murnaghan, 2013), or ALSO (Advanced Life Support in Obstetrics) (American Academy of Family Physicians, 2020).

5. *Assessment and feedback:* Develop a formal checklist to use during simulations, integrating procedural and communication skills. Simulation-derived evaluation and debriefing can be an effective way for a preceptor to share best practices with learners.

6. *Evaluation of the simulation:* Create a way for learners to give the teacher feedback about the simulation.

Other Considerations for Simulation-Based Learning

TEACHING BY SIMULATION IN VARIOUS SETTINGS

Both simple and high-fidelity simulations can be used for one-on-one teaching as part of a clinical placement or in a large group setting in a workshop or academic class. When teaching in a group setting, a series of stations can be set up around the room. For example, when teaching a group of beginners the internal exam, stations can be set up starting from a closed and uneffaced cervix and a high presenting part, progressing to full dilation. A workshop that has a variety of clinical skills stations allows learners to focus on areas where they need practice. Learners can move around stations for any of the skills described above, work in pairs, and give each other feedback.

REMOTE LEARNING

During the COVID–19 pandemic, educators in all health professions adapted their approach to include virtual teaching and practising of skills. Learners can be sent instructions and equipment for home practice, integrating medical equipment and homemade models. Many skills like those described in this chapter can be taught remotely, despite teachers' concerns that they can only be taught in person. After a lecture/demonstration presentation online, the teacher can talk and walk through the skill while learners practise at home. For evaluation, learners can submit photo essays or videos of their work.

SIMULATION ON A VIRTUAL REALITY (VR)/AUGMENTED REALITY (AR) PLATFORM

VR is the use of computer enhanced images in custom goggles worn by the user to create a heightened sense of reality in a simulated environment. These goggles, when combined with physical mannequins during an obstetric simulation, may enhance the learners' understanding of the physiologic events during various aspects of childbirth.

Conclusion

In summary, simulation has been used for centuries worldwide to teach learners to assist in childbirth. In recent years, technology has increased the range of simulators available to teachers. In this chapter, we have given examples from the full range of simulation tools available. At the simple, low-fidelity end of this range are creatively modified household objects, which are inexpensive, universally available, and popular with learners. At the complex, expensive, high-fidelity end of this range are programmable, interactive mannequins that can be used to teach and evaluate both learners and teams in their clinical responses to obstetric emergencies. Depending on the resources available to them, teachers can match the simulators they choose to their educational goals. Irrespective of the type of mannequins chosen, simulation is a core element of perinatal care education—and one that promotes creativity, fun, and team-building while optimizing learners' acquisition of the knowledge and skills needed to assist in safe childbirth.

REFERENCES

Abdelrahman, A., & Murnaghan, M. (2013). Practical obstetric multi-professional training course. British Medical Journal, 2013;346:e8561

American Academy of Family Physicians (2021). Advanced life support in obstetrics (ALSO). American Academy of Family Physicians. https://www.aafp.org/cme/programs/also.html

Andrighetti, T.P., Knestrick, J.M., Marowitz, A., Martin, C., & Engstrom, J.L. (2012). Shoulder dystocia and postpartum hemorrhage simulations: Student confidence in managing these complications. Journal of Midwifery & Women's Health, 57(1), 55-60. doi:10.1111/j.1542-2011.2011.00085.x

Bambini, D. (2016). Writing a simulation scenario: A step-by-step guide. AACN Advanced Critical Care, 27(1), 62-70. doi:10.4037/aacnacc2016986

Bergh, A., Baloyi, S., & Pattinson, R. (2015). What is the impact of multi-professional emergency obstetric and neonatal care training? Best Practice & Research. Clinical Obstetrics & Gynecology, 29(8), 1028-1043. https://doi.org/10.1016/j.bpobgyn.2015.03.017

Blom, K., Iancu, A., Lee, K., Tai, M. (2022) Managing Obstetrical Trauma- Perineal suturing model. Retrieved from https://resourcelibrary.stfm.org/viewdocument/managing-obstetrical-trauma-3?CommunityKey=2751b51d-483f-45e2-81de-4faced0a290a&tab=librarydocuments

Burns, E.S., Duff, M., Leggett, J., & Schmied, V. (2020). Emergency scenarios in maternity: An exploratory study of a midwifery and medical student simulation based learning collaboration. Women and Birth: Journal of the Australian College of Midwives, 34(6), 563-569. doi:10.1016/j.wombi.2020.10.005

Canadian Association of Midwives. (2021). Canadian Emergency Skills Programs. Retrieved at https://canadianmidwives.org/emergency-skills/

Cant, R.P. (2010). Simulation-based learning in nurse education: systematic review. 66(1). Journal of Advanced Nursing, 66(1), 3-15.

Carty, E. (2010). Educating Midwives with the World's First Simulator: Madame du Coudray's Eighteenth Century Mannequin. Canadian Journal of Midwifery Research and Practice. 9, Retrieved at https://www.cjmrp.com/articles/volume-9-2010/educating-midwives-with-the-world-s-first-simulator-madame-du-coudray-s-eighteenth-century-mannequin

Cooper, S., Cant, R., Porter, J., Bogossian, F., McKenna, L., Brady, S., & Fox-Young, S. (2012). Simulation-based learning in midwifery education: A systematic review. Women and Birth: Journal of the Australian College of Midwives, 25(2), 64-78. doi:10.1016/j.wombi.2011.03.004

Costiuc, N. (2021). How Much Does a Human Patient Simulator Cost? Retrieved from https://www.healthysimulation.com/30911/human-patient-simulator-cost/

Deering, S., & Rowland, J. (2013). Obstetric emergency simulation. Seminars in Perinatology, 37(3), 179-188. doi: 10.1053/j.semperi.2013.02.010

Draycott, T., Collins, K., Crofts, J., Siassakos, D., Winter, C., Weiner, C., & Donald, F. (2015). Myths and realities of training in obstetric emergencies. Best Practice & Research. Clinical Obstetrics & Gynecology, 29(8), 1067-1076. https://doi.org/10.1016/j.bpobgyn.2015.07.003

Dziegnel, A. (2016). How to Make a Yarn Rope. BabbleDabbleDo. Retrieved at https://babbled-abbledo.com/yarn-craft-idea-make-yarn-rope/

Ennen, C.S., & Satin, A.J. (2010). Training and assessment in obstetrics: The role of simulation: Training, education and assessment. Best Practice & Research. Clinical Obstetrics & Gynecology, 24(6), 747-758.

Finan, E., Bismilla, Z., Whyte, H.E., Leblanc, V., McNamara, P.J. (2012). High-fidelity simulator technology may not be superior to traditional low-fidelity equipment for neonatal resuscitation training. Journal of Perinatolology, 32, 287–92. https://doi.org/10.1038/jp.2011.96

Fox-Young, S., Brady, S., Brealey, W., Cooper, S., McKenna, L., Hall, H., & Bogossian, F. (2012). The perspectives of Australian midwifery academics on barriers and enablers for simulation in midwifery education in Australia: A focus group study. Midwifery, 28(4), 435-441. https://doi.org/10.1016/j.midw.2011.07.005

Fransen, A.F., van de Ven, J., Banga, F.R., Mol, B.W.J., & Oei, S.G. (2020). Multi-professional simulation-based team training in obstetric emergencies for improving patient outcomes and trainees' performance. Cochrane Database of Systematic Reviews, 12, CD011545-CD011545. doi:10.1002/14651858.CD011545.pub2

Garber, A., Posner, G., El-Chaar, D., & Mitchell, T. (2013). Simulation-based education in obstetrics and gynaecology training in Canada. Journal of Obstetrics and Gynaecology Canada, 35(11), 975-976. doi:10.1016/S1701-2163(15)30782-9

Gardner, R., & Raemer, D. (2008). Simulation in obstetrics and gynecology. Obstetrics and Gynecology Clinics of North America, 35, 97-127.

Garvey, A.A., & Dempsey, E.M. (2020). Simulation in neonatal resuscitation. Frontiers in Pediatrics, 8, 59-59. https://doi.org/10.3389/fped.2020.00059

Hammond, J. (2014). Perineal Repair. Schulich School of Medicine Western University Retrieved from https://www.youtube.com/watch?v=teukCoeaDqo

Harrington, D.W. (2021). Designing a Simulation Scenario. StatPearls Publishing. Retrieved at https://www.statpearls.com/ArticleLibrary/viewarticle/63807

Johannsson, H., Ayida, G., & Sadler, C. (2005). Faking it? Simulation in the training of obstetricians and gynaecologists. Current Opinion in Obstetrics & Gynecology, 17(6), 557-561. doi: 10.1097/01.gco.0000188726.45998.97

Lai, W. (2004). Instructions for the paper pelvis. Retrieved at https://weishinlai.tripod.com/pelvis/

Laporte, V. (2012). Perineal Repair: Yellow sponge simulator 2nd degree tear. University of Michigan. Retrieved from https://www.youtube.com/watch?v=R4o4KSY4MMY

Lendahls, L., Oscarsson, M.G. (2017). Midwifery students' experiences of simulation and skills training. Nurse Education Today, 50, 12-16.

Massoth, C., Röder, H., Ohlenburg, H., Hessler, M., Zarbock, A., Pöpping, D.M., & Wenk, M. (2019). High-fidelity is not superior to low-fidelity simulation but leads to overconfidence in medical students. BMC Medical Education, 19(1), 29-29. https://doi.org/10.1186/s12909-019-1464-7

Merien, A.E., van de Ven, J., Mol, B.W., Houterman, S. & Oei S.G. (2010 May). Multidisciplinary team training in a simulation setting for acute obstetric emergencies: a systematic review. Obstetrics and Gynecology, 115(5),1021-31.

McLaughlin, S., Fitch, M., Goyal, D., Hayden, E., Kauh, C., Laack, T., Nowicki, T., Okuda, Y., Palm, K., Pozner, C.N., Vozenilek, J., Wang, E., & Gordon, J.A. (2008). Simulation in graduate medical education: A review for emergency medicine. Academic Emergency Medicine, 15(11), 1117-1129. doi: 10.1111/j.1553-2712.2008.00188.x

Okuda, Y., Bryson, E.O., DeMaria, S.J., Jacobson, L., Quinones, J., Shen, B. & Levine, A.I. (2009 Aug) The utility of simulation in medical education: what is the evidence? Mt Sinai Journal, 76(4), 330-43.

Reszel, J., Weiss, D., Sprague, A.E., Fell, D.B., Dunn, S., Walker, M.C. & Peterson, W.E. (2019). A mixed-methods evaluation of the MOREob program in Ontario hospitals: Participant knowledge, organizational culture, and experiences. BioMed Central Health Services Research, 19(1), 460-460. doi:10.1186/s12913-019-4224-9

Satin, A.J. (2018). Simulation in Obstetrics. Obstetrics and Gynecology, 132(1), 199–209. https://doi.org/10.1097/AOG.0000000000002682

Ting, H. (2020) How to repair a 2nd degree perineal tear: a suturing workshop. University of British Columbia Medicine. Retrieved from https://www.youtube.com/watch?v=86YBAjim_Rw

Van Wagner, V. & Chu, H. (2012) Using simple simulation to teach midwifery skills, 11(1), 20-34. Retrieved at https://www.cjmrp.com/files/v11n1-van-wagner-simulation.pdf.

Weiner, C., Samuelson, L., Collins, L., & Satterwhite, C. (2014). 61: 5-year experience with PROMP (Practical obstetric multidisciplinary training) reveals sustained and progressive improvements in obstetric outcomes at a US hospital. American Journal of Obstetrics and Gynecology, 210(1), S40-S40. doi:10.1016/j.ajog.2013.10.094

Windrim, R., Ehman, W., Carson, G.D., Kollesh, L., & Milne, K. (2006). The ALARM course: 10 years of continuing professional development in intrapartum care and risk management in Canada. Journal of Obstetrics and Gynaecology Canada, 28(7), 600-602. doi: 10.1016/S1701-2163(16)32212-5

Chapter 5

TEACHING LEARNERS ABOUT BREASTFEEDING

Natalie Morson, Amanda Pendergrast, Kate Snead

Dr. Joy is a new family physician with a comprehensive practice that includes perinatal care. She enjoys teaching medical students and residents and has learners working with her most days of the week. After approximately a year of practice and observation of several learner-patient encounters both in her clinic and on the postpartum floor, Dr. Joy recognizes what little experience her learners have in assisting new mothers and infants with breastfeeding and grows concerned with their lack of breastfeeding medicine knowledge overall. Knowing how important breastfeeding is for maternal and infant health outcomes, she is worried these learners will not be well prepared to help with breastfeeding education and troubleshooting challenging cases once out in practice. She feels this gap in learning is not unique to her educational institution and knows there are several studies that show breastfeeding education has not been well-established for medical learners in a variety of institutions (Pound et al., 2014; Chuisano & Anderson, 2019; Rodriguez & Shattuck, 2017).

Dr. Joy speaks with several colleagues, who all agree this is an educational gap in medical training, and they work together to come up with some ideas to address this need. Recognizing there are no dedicated breastfeeding-only learning opportunities, Dr. Joy and her colleagues create a document of teaching strategies they can use to incorporate breastfeeding education both in an opportunistic manner and as a purposeful plan during their clinical everyday teaching.

Teaching Using Patient Encounters

Clinical opportunities for teaching breastfeeding can happen in various settings including the outpatient clinic (during prenatal, postpartum, or well-baby visits), the home or in the hospital or birthing centre.

UNDERSTANDING AND PREPARING YOUR LEARNER

Regardless of the teaching setting, it is important to understand the learner's present state of knowledge as well as their learning goals. Assess their comfort and experience with infants and breastfeeding parents to gauge the level of independence you should accord them. They should identify any gaps they recognize in their knowledge or previous training. This will help tailor their education to their needs.

Most medical learners are inexperienced in breastfeeding medicine and not confident in their clinical skills in this area (Pound et al., 2014). Some, however, will have more experience with breastfeeding—either from previous clinical encounters or from personal experience. No matter their previous experience, it is important to assess their attitude toward breastfeeding.

Example:

You are working with a medical student in your family medicine clinic. Your clinic schedule includes a few well-baby visits, including a newborn check. When you discuss this case with your student, she conveys that she has very little experience with newborns and is not comfortable holding a baby. She is very nervous about having to discuss breastfeeding with the baby's mother.

In this scenario, the following tips may be helpful in preparing an inexperienced learner for the encounter:

- **Demonstrate baby-holding techniques using a doll.** It can be very useful to have dolls available in the clinic to demonstrate baby-holding. Use a child's toy or a doll commercially available for breastfeeding teaching (see Appendix A). This provides learners with the opportunity to practise holding a newborn. For example, you might demonstrate how to pick up the doll as though it were a real baby, describing how you provide support to the head and neck and showing the learner where to place their hands to feel secure carrying a newborn.

- **Prepare learners for common issues that arise.** If time permits, before the start of clinic or in a gap between encounters, it can be helpful to prime the learner with some of the common issues and questions that arise during early newborn visits.

- **Provide educational handouts directed at parents to the learner.** If the learner has not encountered many newborns in their training, providing educational handouts designed for parents can help provide context. These handouts may be given to patients at prenatal classes, breastfeeding classes, or in the postpartum ward. These handouts can help guide the learner when teaching to new parents during the critical first few weeks. Examples of parent guides can be found in Appendix C.

Example:

You are supervising a first-year family medicine resident whose partner has just delivered a healthy baby girl. He has just returned to work after a short paternity leave. While observing his encounter with a new mother and her 6-day-old infant, you notice that he makes a few comments, such as "Isn't breastfeeding wonderful?" and "My partner really enjoys breastfeeding our daughter." He does an excellent job taking a full breastfeeding history, including ascertaining whether the mother's milk has come in, asking about frequency of feeds, and determining appropriate urine output and bowel movement frequency. He even offers to observe a breastfeeding session to assess the latch.

Here are a few tips that can be helpful when dealing with more experienced learners:

- **Evaluate potential impact of learners' prior experiences.** Learners who have personal experiences with breastfeeding may have a biased perspective on what a typical breastfeeding experience will look like. Someone who had a very positive personal experience may erroneously assume that all breastfeeding journeys are smooth. This can result in the type of comments illustrated in the case above, which can leave a patient feeling insecure or inadequate if they are struggling or not enjoying breastfeeding. Conversely, a learner who struggled to breastfeed their own children (or whose partner struggled) may approach parents and babies with an expectation of difficulty that may have a negative impact on patient experience. It is important to help learners identify any biases they may bring into the patient encounter.

- **Take the opportunity to teach at a higher level.** When learners have a good understanding of the basics of breastfeeding, you can take the opportunity to teach them some more advanced information and skills. Some of the higher-level topics that you can tackle in this scenario include . . .

  - Practising additional breastfeeding holds with dolls
  - Counselling on-hand expression and practical experience with breast models
  - The use of a breast pump
  - When and how to utilize lactation aids
  - Ankyloglossia and the role of frenotomies

See Appendix C for some online resources that can be helpful for teaching these topics.

TEACHING DURING WELL-BABY VISITS

The most common place that breastfeeding teaching can happen is during well-baby visits. This can provide an opportunity to discuss the normal trajectory of breastfeeding, common challenges that arise, and demonstrate how to properly assess and correct a latch.

Example:

You are working with a first-year family medicine resident in your family medicine clinic. He has just completed a history on a 3-day old baby who is in the office for a weight check. The mother is reporting significant nipple pain with breastfeeding and is worried about the baby having lost 7.5 percent of his birth weight. The resident is wondering if formula should be used as supplementation.

You can use this opportunity to help the resident learn how to assess breastfeeding in the first days of life.

Here are some tips that will help in this scenario:

- **Provide a template to guide breastfeeding history taking.** New learners are often overwhelmed by the questions they need to ask when taking a breastfeeding history. It can be helpful to provide a basic template they can work from. This will prompt them to ask the key questions. Then, you can work together to put the information together to form your assessment. See Appendix D for a sample template. Learners can also be encouraged to use published evidence-based tools, such as the Newfoundland and Labrador Physician Breastfeeding Toolkit (Pendergast et al., 2016) or the Rourke Baby Record (Rourke Baby Record, 2020) to prompt the discussion.

- **Observe the encounter directly where possible.** Asking the right questions is just one piece of a successful breastfeeding history. It is equally important to ensure that learners are asking questions in a supportive manner, recognizing that infant feeding can be an emotionally charged issue for new parents. Directly observing these encounters can allow you to provide feedback to learners on things like how they word their questions and their body language (Henry et al., 2013). Learners may become uncomfortable or overwhelmed with questions from new parents (Gary et al., 2017; Dykes, 2006), so it is important to ensure that the teaching environment is supportive and that they are able to ask for help if needed.

- **Guide the learner to comfortably hold and position a newborn.** If the learner has little experience with infants, it can be intimidating for them to perform a physical exam. Ensure they are able to practise positioning a newborn to feed using doll models, eventually progressing to real newborns. For example, if the resident observed a new mother using a cross-cradle hold during an encounter, when debriefing afterward, you may spend a few minutes using a doll to teach the learner about other types of holds, explaining when they might be suggested to a patient. The learner can then practise and demonstrate these holds with the doll.

- **Take the time to model a latch assessment.** Learners are often not confident in their ability to assess an effective breastfeeding latch. Asking the lactating parent to latch the baby during the encounter can provide an opportunity to simultaneously teach the parents how to identify a successful latch and provide the learner with an approach to assessing a successful latch and correcting a painful one. Other tools may be used to reinforce the learning, such as videos (see Appendix B). This will also help to reinforce that this skill is within the scope of practice of a family physician, and that it does not require referral to a lactation consultant. In future encounters, you can encourage the learner to perform the latch assessment independently, observing and providing them with feedback.

- **Debrief after the encounter.** Learners will often have questions they are embarrassed to ask with the patient in the room. It is important to provide a safe space for this after patient encounters. This will also give you an opportunity to provide some information on topics like the expected course of infant weight gain and breastmilk production in the first weeks of life. This time can also be used to develop a plan for the next encounter of this kind.

- **Address how gender may impact the patient encounter**. It is important for you, as a teacher, to acknowledge how the perceived gender of the learner may influence the comfort level of both the patient and the learner during a breastfeeding encounter. The impact this can have on the outcome of the therapeutic relationship may range from minimal (i.e., a concern for neither person involved) to being a significant barrier to the interaction. Being aware of this and sensitive to the needs of your patient and your learner will make you a more supportive and effective teacher. Letting your patients know that a learner (of any gender) may be present during visits can help answer their questions, alleviate their apprehension, and identify those patients with whom a learner may not be appropriate.

TEACHING DURING PRENATAL VISITS

Prenatal visits also present an opportunity to teach important concepts regarding infant feeding. Just as these visits can set the stage for success with parents, they can provide a good foundation for the medical learner.

Example:

A 2nd-year family medicine resident is meeting a new prenatal patient. She takes a full history and completes a physical exam. She returns to review the case with you and says she is uncertain as to how to discuss the patient's intentions for newborn feeding or how to perform a breast assessment.

Here are a few suggestions that can be used during prenatal visits to encourage learning about breastfeeding:

- **Model ways to open the discussion about infant feeding.** Learners are often taught the benefits of breastfeeding but not how to discuss preferred infant feeding in a patient-centred manner. Teaching the learner how to ask this question in an open-ended, non-judgmental way is essential. Provide guidance to introduce the topic of infant feeding with the parents. It can be helpful to provide a scripted statement or question to open the discussion, such as, "Have you thought about how you want to feed your baby?" or "Are you hoping to breastfeed or bottle-feed your baby?" Asking the right questions in the right way is very important. Direct observation of the learner speaking with expectant parents can be helpful. This skill can also be practised through roleplay.

- **Prepare and guide the learner to perform breast examinations.** Learners are often hesitant to discuss pregnancy-related breast changes with patients and may be uncomfortable performing breast exams (regardless of their gender). Assess their current comfort level, then offer to start by modelling the exam and discussion first. Provide tips on how to ensure they are professional in performing this sensitive exam, including in performing proper draping and ensuring the patient feels at ease. Ensure the learner is aware of normal and abnormal findings. During the following prenatal exam, you could have the learner demonstrate this skill under supervision so that they feel supported. Then, you can slowly increase the level of independence granted them as they gain familiarity and confidence. Do be sure, however, to discuss the appropriate use of chaperones for sensitive exams.

- **Use breast models for teaching.** Have a few breast models available in your clinic to use for teaching either in preparing for a specific patient encounter or during a free moment during the day. These models can be as simple as a knitted breast with a bean bag inside or a foam breast-shaped stress ball (see Appendix A). The advantage of using a breast model is that you can explicitly discuss hand placement, the appropriate pressure to apply, and how to teach these skills to patients in a helpful and respectful manner.

- **Use short educational videos to solidify skills.** It may be difficult for a learner to visualize what hand expression and milk ejection looks like if they have had minimal exposure during their training or no personal experience with breastfeeding. A short educational video (Appendix B) may be helpful for them to understand how the breast changes during pregnancy, breast anatomy that may hinder lactation, and how to teach hand expression.

TEACHING DURING INTRAPARTUM CARE

There is often downtime in the labour and delivery ward, during which teaching opportunities may arise. This can be a great opportunity to teach learners about how to support breastfeeding initiation.

Example:

You are attending a delivery with a 1st-year family medicine resident who has a keen interest in perinatal care and breastfeeding. The patient is nearing the second stage and is stable. You and the resident work on the chart notes. Before going into the patient room to commence pushing, you discuss how you as a team will manage the delivery and what comes after. This can be a useful time to discuss how to approach breastfeeding in the first hours of life and the role that the labour and delivery team can play in a successful start to breastfeeding.

The important topics to cover with a learner in this area include . . .

- **The importance of the "golden hour."** It is important to inquire as to the previous experiences of the learner, specifically with regard to their knowledge around breastfeeding in the first hour after delivery, also known as the "golden hour." Many learners are not familiar with this concept. Explain how some routine practices are meant to support the initiation of breastfeeding, including facilitating uninterrupted skin-to-skin contact immediately after birth and waiting to do non-essential procedures (such as weighing the baby and the first newborn exam—and how one might consider performing the first newborn exam while baby is skin-to-skin with the parent) (Feldman-Winter et al., 2016; World Health Organization 2021). If time permits, you can also consider using some video resources to demonstrate proper latch techniques (Appendix B).

- **The learner's knowledge of institution-specific practices.** Discuss the breastfeeding supports available in your institution and identify how common practices may support or impede breastfeeding success. Encourage the learner to consider special circumstances, such as premature delivery or Caesarean section and how to support breastfeeding in these cases. Some institutions may be more amenable to employing skin-to-skin in these instances, others might require more advocacy on the part of the family physician. For institutions where policy dictates non-skin-to-skin practices, consider other ways to enhance breastfeeding, such as having the partner employ skin-to-skin during a Caesarean section if the mother is unable or using a breast pump after a premature delivery.

- **Modelling hands-on experience.** The "golden hour" can be an excellent opportunity to model the role of the family physician in supporting breastfeeding. Allow the learner to observe you help the mother latch the baby for the first time. Demonstrate how to latch the baby and how a latch should look. If the learner is experienced, they can assist. To allow further development of knowledge and skill, consider recommending the learner spend time with the nurses or lactation consultants to hone their skills. Consider asking the learner to review breastfeeding videos (Appendix B) after the patient encounter to support their learning.

This role-modelling will not only help in skill development—it will also reinforce that this is an important part of one's role as a perinatal care provider.

- **Teaching during the newborn examination.** The first newborn exam is often done in the delivery room and can provide an opportunity for some important teaching. First of all, it is an opportunity for learners to gain confidence in holding and positioning a newborn. It can also be an opportunity to identify any physical issues that might impact breastfeeding. In particular, if a tongue tie is noted, this can be an opportunity to discuss how this may impact feeding and the potential role for a frenotomy to improve latch.

TEACHING IN THE POSTPARTUM WARD

Example:

You round on the postpartum floor to assess a newborn you delivered last night. A 1st-year family medicine resident accompanies you on the rounds. She has personal experience, as she recently returned from parental leave and continues to breastfeed her daughter. After assessing a first-time mother and baby, she returns to review the case. The new mother wants to breastfeed, but her milk does not come in at 24 hours and she experiences nipple pain. The resident encourages her to continue. However, the mother wants to add formula supplementation. The resident is not sure how to proceed.

You enter the patient's room with the learner. The patient is tearful, as she expected breastfeeding to be natural and easy. She understands the benefits of breastfeeding but is fearful her baby is hungry. She had never thought that breastfeeding would be more painful than labour. She wants to stop breastfeeding. You examine her breasts and notice nipple abrasions. You discuss her goals with infant feeding and make a plan to help her reach them. You assure her that the most important point is that her baby gets fed and that you will help her whether she continues to breastfeed or not.

The following tips may help a learner feel more comfortable assessing newborns and their birthing parents.

- **Round with the learner.** This is a valuable opportunity to model conversations about breastfeeding with new parents. For the inexperienced learner, watching these encounters can help them understand the natural course of breastfeeding in the first days as well as feel more comfortable approaching these conversations. Even with learners who breastfed their own children, observing latches and breastfeeding holds provides the opportunity to learn how patients' situations may differ from the learner's personal experience. Reassure the learner that not all patients will breastfeed when they leave the postpartum ward. Be an advocate for your patient and ensure there are adequate supports available.

- **Enlist the expertise of nursing and lactation consultant colleagues.** There are often many sources of support in the hospital for breastfeeding parents. As a result, there are many opportunities for learners to enhance their breastfeeding knowledge. If breastfeeding classes are offered, learners should be encouraged to attend. If a colleague has several patients in hospital, the learner may accompany them on rounds. For those wishing for more experience, a morning in the postpartum ward with the postpartum nurses may be arranged. The learners can further develop their skills in assisting with latch and teaching breastfeeding holds. Finally, if the learner is interested in viewing more challenging cases, they could spend time with the lactation consultant on inpatient and outpatient consults or arrange to shadow a public health nurse on a postpartum home visit.

Other Teaching Strategies

TEACHING FROM VIDEO REVIEW AND CHART REVIEW

Using video technology is an effective way to participate in direct observation of the learner (Rubenstein & Talbot, 2019). Try to set aside time for video or chart review focused on breastfeeding knowledge and hands-on skills.

Example:

You are working with a 2nd-year family medicine resident who is experienced in breastfeeding education. She has counselled a patient at 38 weeks' gestation on the golden hour of breastfeeding, as well as answered questions about colostrum and hand expression. The learner obtained consent from the patient to videotape the interview. During your lunch hour, you book time with the learner to review the video.

Here is how you might approach teaching learners in this way:

- **Observe an entire interview.** To ensure the learner is conducting a patient-centred interview, an entire learner-patient encounter may be watched. As breastfeeding can be a sensitive topic, watching the learner's initial approach, the manner in which they ask questions, and the tone of the interview can be as important as the content of what they say. Any gaps in knowledge around breastfeeding may be identified and corrected. The preceptor can check for learners' assessment of other factors that support breastfeeding, such as inquiring about partner support and return to work.

- **Choose specific skills to observe and provide feedback.** Alternatively, the preceptor may choose select areas to review. This might include viewing the beginning of the interview to see how the learner broaches the topic of breastfeeding and how they ask for consent. They might instead observe the end of the interview to see how the plan is summarized with the patient, or observe a learner demonstrating a specific skill on a model to a patient, such as hand expression.

- **Use chart review and chart-stimulated recall to identify gaps in knowledge.** The learner or preceptor can choose a patient encounter to review. The patient encounter may be a prenatal or postpartum visit. The review may include history taking, decision-making, communication, diagnosis, and documentation related to breastfeeding (Schipper & Ross, 2010). If required, the learner can be supplied with evidence-based material for further learning. See examples in Appendix C.

- **Consider using short didactic presentations.** It can be helpful to have a repository of patient cases or short presentations organized and filed for easy access at any time (e.g., on your laptop, cellphone, or a booklet in your lab coat). These presentations can focus both on important basic topics that you want to teach but that may not be encountered organically in patient encounters and more advanced topics (e.g., mastitis, low breastmilk supply, domperidone prescribing, weaning, medication safety, pumping and storage). The selection of what to teach on any given day should be based on the educational goals your learner has for their rotation, their interests, and any knowledge gaps they have.

TEACHING THROUGH WORKSHOPS

Breastfeeding workshops are an excellent way to provide education for a larger group of learners. Group learning can be an opportunity for students to establish a foundation of basic knowledge or reinforce their previous learning and allow for them to practise and refine their skills. Workshops are meant to act as a supplement to direct patient encounters.

The following are some tips for planning your workshop:

- **Involve colleagues from complementary professions.** Interprofessional collaboration for teaching breastfeeding can enrich the learning experience for students and prove to be invaluable. For example, you might invite a local lactation consultant and a postpartum nurse educator to help facilitate small group breakout sessions to teach breastmilk hand expression. They can assist the small groups by giving instruction, providing feedback regarding technique, and answering questions as they arise. Supporting breastfeeding involves many members of the healthcare team, and this can be a good opportunity to model interprofessional collaboration.

- **Keep the groups small.** Plan for small groups—typically, six to ten learners is an ideal. If you are conducting a larger group session on breastfeeding, plan opportunities to break out into smaller groups for discussion and hands-on practice. Even numbers of participants will help learners pair up for roleplaying clinician and patient.

- **Roleplay.** Roleplay can be useful for practising interviewing techniques or practical skills. Simulation during a workshop provides a safe space for learning breastfeeding-related skills and the freedom for learners to ask questions they might not typically feel comfortable inquiring about in front of real patients. For example, workshop participants can practise how they might teach hand expression of breastmilk to their patients. They can work on hand placement and appropriate pressure application on model breasts. Other skills to roleplay might include holding and positioning a baby with a doll, teaching a patient's partner how to set up and utilize a lactation aid, and walking through using a breast pump with a first-time lactating parent (see Appendix A).

Learners can also practise interviewing and counselling techniques. These might include discussing emotionally charged topics, such as preferred infant feeding methods, where one person plays the role of the physician and the other acts as a soon-to-be parent in a prenatal appointment.

- **Recognize that hands-on experience is valuable to learners.** When planning your teaching in a group setting, whether a lecture or workshop, it is important to recognize the value of hands-on learning to the learner. Plan for sufficient time in the workshop for learners to handle and practise using breastfeeding equipment—lactation aids, breast pumps, and so forth—so they will be more confident and knowledgeable when translating this to an in-person encounter with a patient (Feldman-Winter et al., 2010).

- **Create a panel of experts.** Invite a group of experts to participate in a question-and-answer panel. Ideally, this would be at the end of your workshop, after attendees have been introduced to all the material and you have had the opportunity to collect questions. The panel might include interprofessional colleagues (lactation consultants, midwives, nurses, other family physicians, pediatricians) and might possibly also include patients with varying experiences with breastfeeding. There are many different options for how to conduct a panel discussion, but they usually start with each panellist introducing themselves. After introductions, some panellists may share their "story" with breastfeeding, and others may have clinical "pearls" or tips on working with new parents and babies. And of course, ensure there is ample time for attendees to ask the panel questions. Ensure that either your or someone else who is not on the panel is designated as the moderator to track time, watch for raised hands in the group for questions, and provide clarification as needed when answers are provided.

- **Consider case-based teaching.** For any content-based components of your workshop, use cases to illustrate key points. These may help learners stay engaged in the topic and generate more interaction between the workshop attendees (Volpe Holmes et al., 2012).

  For example, when seeing a breastfeeding patient with an erythematous and painful breast, your learner might be more apt at recalling your story of diagnosing and treating "Kristen, who had sore and cracked nipples when feeding her new baby girl" versus a generic talk on mastitis. Include photos to show how similar diagnoses may present in different patients to help ingrain recall.

- **Using videos for teaching.** Videos can be a very useful tool during your workshop. They are especially helpful for demonstrating the difference between a good and poor latch and how to look for suck-and-swallow. However, if using videos (such as the ones in Appendix B), take time to pause the video, ask the learners questions as to what they are seeing, and point out important positions, features, and moments you want them to pay attention to. This will help engage the learner while they watch the video, instead of having them passively take in the information.

- **Provide take-home materials from the workshop.** Consider providing the learners with written materials at the end of the lecture or workshop for them to refer to when working with patients in their clinical practice. These may come in the form of lecture slides, handouts, or evidence-based toolkits. Examples can be found at the end of this chapter.

E-LEARNING

There are a number of scenarios where e-learning can support and augment in-person clinical learning around breastfeeding. Some clinical environments do not provide enough clinical breastfeeding encounters for learners. In other circumstances, learners have downtime when on call or are looking for additional learning experiences to supplement their clinical ones. In both these scenarios, asynchronous e-learning can be a useful educational tool.

The following are publicly available online modules that can be used either for self-directed learning or as part of a breastfeeding curriculum.

- City of Toronto Breastfeeding E-Learning Modules

  https://www.toronto.ca/community-people/health-wellness-care/information-for-healthcare-professionals/maternal-child-health-info-for-doctors/breastfeeding/breastfeeding-e-learning-modules/

- Children's Hospital of Eastern Ontario Pediatric Teaching Files
  - https://www.cheo.on.ca/en/resources/TongueTie/story_html5.html
  - https://www.cheo.on.ca/en/resources/FeedingDifficulties/story_html5.html
  - https://www.cheo.on.ca/en/resources/JaundicedInfant/story_html5.html

Appendix A:
Equipment Suggestions for Breastfeeding Teaching

Equipment	Options	Advantages	Limitations	Approximate Cost*
Dolls - for teaching breastfeeding holds/ newborn care	Newborn teaching doll (from a medical supply company such as Birth Supplies Canada Inc., Laerdal, etc.)	- Realistic - Weighted - Easy to clean - Open-mouthed - Durable - Variety of skin colours	- Higher cost	$150 CAD per doll
	Any children's baby doll (purchased/ donated)	- Lower cost	- May contain fabric (not ideal for cleaning between uses) - Less realistic	$0-50 CAD per doll
Breast models - for teaching hand expression	Foam breasts (breast-shaped stress balls)	- Low cost - Easy to clean	- No variability in sizes of breasts, areolas, or nipples	$2 CAD per breast
	Knitted/ crocheted breast models (purchased or made)	- Can be customized (size/shape)	- Higher cost - Time-consuming to make - Cannot be disinfected	$20 CAD per breast (purchased) $10 CAD (homemade)
Breast Pump - for demonstrating its use, reviewing flange sizes	- Old/used pump - Borrowed from lactation clinic			Variable
Lactation Simulator	Available online	Excellent for hands-on teaching (latch, holds, hand expression, etc.)	Expensive	$200-$1500 CAD

*PLEASE NOTE THESE ARE ROUGH ESTIMATES AS OF 2022 AND WILL VARY BASED ON LOCATION, AVAILABILITY, QUANTITY, SHIPPING, ETC.

Appendix B:
Video Suggestions for Breastfeeding Teaching

- Breastmilk Hand Expression

  - www.globalhealthmedia.org

    - Click "Our Videos"
    - Click "Small Baby"
    - Click "How to Express Your First Milk"

      - Key content: 1:00–4:30

  https://globalhealthmedia.org/portfolio-items/how-to-express-your-first-milk/?portfolioCats=191%2C94%2C13%2C23%2C65

- Breastfeeding Latch

  - www.globalhealthmedia.org

    - Click "Our Videos"
    - Click "Breastfeeding"
    - Click "Attaching Your Baby at the Breast"

      - Key content: 0:31–9:42

  https://globalhealthmedia.org/portfolio-items/attaching-your-baby-at-the-breast/?portfolioCats=191%2C94%2C13%2C23%2C65

- Early Initiation of Breastfeeding (the "golden hour")

  - www.globalhealthmedia.org

    - Click "Our Videos"
    - Click "Breastfeeding"
    - Click "Early Initiation of Breastfeeding"

      - Key content: 6:20–8:14

  https://med.stanford.edu/newborns/professional-education/breastfeeding/early-initiation-of-breastfeeding.html

Appendix C:
Helpful Resources for Breastfeeding Teaching

- Best Start by Nexus Sante: Breastfeeding

  - www.beststart.org

    - Click "Resources"
    - Click "Breastfeeding"

      · Click: "Breastfeeding: Guidelines for Consultants"

https://resources.beststart.org/product/b03e-breastfeeding-guidelines-for-consultants/

      · Click "My Breastfeeding Guide"

https://resources.beststart.org/product/b20e-my-breastfeeding-guide-booklet/

      · Click "Signs That Feeding is Going Well"

https://resources.beststart.org/product/b02e-signs-feeding-going-well/

- City of Toronto: Learning to Breastfeed

  - www.toronto.ca

    - Search "Learning to Breastfeed"

https://www.toronto.ca/community-people/children-parenting/pregnancy-and-parenting/breastfeeding/breastfeeding-your-baby/learning-to-breastfeed/

- Baby-Friendly Newfoundland and Labrador: The Physician's Breastfeeding Toolkit: Quick Reference Guide

  - www.babyfriendlynl.ca

    - Click "For Health Care Professionals"
    - Click "Physician's Toolkit Quick Reference Guide"

https://babyfriendlynl.ca/app/uploads/2019/01/BFToolkitQuick Reference.pdf

Appendix D:
Sample Clinical Note Template for
EMR to Assess Infant Feeding

1. Age of infant: __

2. Birth weight: __ g

3. Current weight: __ g

   – If below birth weight: __ % weight loss
   – If gaining weight, weight gain since last visit: __ g/day

4. Mode of feeding: exclusive breastfeeding / exclusive pumped breastmilk / mix of breast and bottle or lactation aid (pumped milk/formula) / exclusive formula

5. Frequency of feeding: -- q ___ hours

6. Both breasts at each feed? yes / no

7. Length of each feed: __ min/breast

8. Baby waking themselves for feeds? yes / no

9. Baby seems satisfied after each feed? yes / no

10. Effective latch? yes / no

    If no, details: _____

11. Painful latch? yes / no

    If yes, details: _____

12. Lactation consultant involved? yes / no

    If yes, details: _____

13. Number of wet diapers per twenty-four-hour period: __

14. Stool output:

    – Number of diapers per twenty-four-hour period: __
    – Colour: _____

REFERENCES

Best Start by Nexus Sante. (2020). Breastfeeding: Guidelines for consultants. Best Start by Nexus Sante. https://resources.beststart.org/product/b03e-breastfeeding-guidelines-for-consultants/

Best Start by Nexus Sante. (2020). My breastfeeding guide. Best Start by Nexus Sante. https://resources.beststart.org/product/b20e-my-breastfeeding-guide-booklet/

Best Start by Nexus Sante. (2020). Signs that feeding is going well. Retrieved March 03, 2021, from https://resources.beststart.org/product/b02e-signs-feeding-going-well/

Chuisano, S.A., & Anderson, O.S. (2019). Assessing application-based breastfeeding education for physicians and nurses: A coping review. Journal of Human Lactation, 36(4), 699-709.

Dabson, A.M., Magin, P.J., & Heading, G. (2014). Medical students' experiences learning intimate physical examination skills: a qualitative study. BioMed Central Medical Education, 14, 39. https://doi.org/10.1186/1472-6920-14-39

Dykes, F. (2006). The education of health practitioners supporting breastfeeding women: time for critical reflection. Maternal and Child Nutrition, 2(4), 204-216.

Feldman-Winter, L., Barone, L., Milcarek, B., Hunter, K., Meek, J., Morton, J., Williams, T., Naylor, A., & Lawrence, R.A. (2010). Residency curriculum improved breastfeeding care. Pediatrics, 126(2), 289-297.

Feldman-Winter, L., & Goldsmith, J.P. (2016). Safe sleep and skin-to-skin care in the neonatal period for healthy term newborns. Pediatrics, 138(3), e20161889.

Gary, A., Birmingham, E., & Jones, L. (2017). Improving breastfeeding medicine in undergraduate medical education: A student survey and extensive curriculum review with suggestions for improvement. Education Health (Abingdon), 30(2), 163-168.

Henry, S.G., Holmboe, E.S., & Frankel, R.M. (2013). Evidence-based competencies for improving communication skills in graduate medical education: A review with suggestions for implementation, Medical Teacher, 35, 5, 395-403. doi: 10.3109/0142159X.2013.769677

Pendergast, A., Fox Beer, J., Murphy Goodridge, J., Rudofsky, R., & Bessell, C. (2016). Newfoundland and Labrador Physicians Breastfeeding Toolkit. Retrieved April 19, 2021, from https://babyfriendlynl.ca/support/physicians/

Pound, C.M., Williams, K., Grenon, R., Aglipay, M., & Plint, A.C. (2014). Breastfeeding knowledge, confidence, beliefs, and attitudes of Canadian physicians. Journal of Human Lactation, 30(3), 298-309.

Rodriguez Lien, E., & Shattuck, K. (2017). Breastfeeding education and support services provided to family medicine and obstetrics-gynecology residents. Breastfeeding Medicine, 12(9), 548-553.

Rourke Baby Record. (2020). Retrieved April 19, 2021, from https://www.rourkebabyrecord.ca/rbr2020/default

Rubenstein, W., & Talbot, Y. (2013). Medical Teaching in Ambulatory Care 3rd edition. University of Toronto Press.

Schipper, S., & Ross, S. (2010). Structured teaching and assessment. A new chart-simulated recall worksheet for family medicine residents. Canadian Family Physician, 56(9), 958-959.

Volpe Holmes, A., Yerdon McLeod, A., Thesing, C., Kramer, S., & Howard, C.R. (2012). Physician breastfeeding education leads to practice changes and improved clinical outcomes. Breastfeeding Medicine, 7(6), 403-408.

World Health Organization. (2021). Ten steps to successful breastfeeding. Retrieved June 9, 2021, from https://www.who.int/activities/promoting-baby-friendly-hospitals/ten-steps-to-successful-breastfeeding

Chapter 6

THE GENERATIONAL DIVIDE: IMPACT ON TEACHING

Erin Bearss, Milena Forte

Dr. Malinda Forss, a family physician and proud member of Gen X, has been practising for fifteen years, and is now taking her career in a new direction by settling in a community with a teaching hospital. She will be working with residents on the labour floor for the first time. While excited about the opportunity to teach, she is anxious about wading into this new environment, particularly with the younger cohort of learners she'll be teaching, who are literally from a different generation. She has signed up for a faculty development workshop on the ABCs of Gens X, Y, and Z for some advice on bridging this generational gap and ensuring her teaching is relevant or "hip to the times."

The Relevance of Generational Theory to Teaching and Learning

The integration and collaboration of different generations in medicine in general and on the labour floor in particular can contribute to diversity and success. It can, however, also present some challenges and result in conflict. The keys to optimizing the advantages and mitigating the potential tensions are to . . .

- Understand the characteristics of generational cohorts
- Appreciate common potential tension points within cohorts

- Engage in deliberate strategies to enhance teaching and learning in the perinatal care environment

Generational Cohorts

"Anything that is in the world when you're born is normal and ordinary and just a natural part of the way the world works.

Anything that's invented between when you're fifteen and thirty-five is new and exciting and revolutionary and you can probably get a career in it.

Anything invented after you're thirty-five is against the natural order of things." *(Adams, 2002)*

A generation is defined as people born and living at approximately the same time with . . .

- Shared life experiences
- Mutual values, beliefs, attitudes, and behaviours (Roberts et al., 2012)

The commonly recognized generations currently encountered in health professions education are Baby Boomers, Generation X, Millennials, and Generation Z.

While it can be helpful to describe the characteristics of each generation, these descriptors are generalizations that may not apply to all members of a cohort, and we caution teachers and learners to be aware of stereotypes and biases.

That being said, what follows are some commonly agreed-upon features of each generation.

BABY BOOMERS (BORN 1945–1964)

- Born post-WWII
- Have a strong work ethic and commitment to their workplace
- Are accustomed to a traditional—and often hierarchical—education style where learners are dependent on the teacher (e.g., didactic lectures)

- Are less tech-savvy than their younger counterparts (Aaron & Levenberg, 2014; Williams et al., 2017)

GEN X (BORN 1965–1980)

- Are independent and self-directed (they often have travelled to and from school on their own at a young age and had a "key necklace," exemplified by the expression "latchkey kids")
- Can be resistant to authority or traditional hierarchical structures
- Recognize the value of work but work to live rather than live to work; work-life balance holds more importance to them
- Are independent, resourceful problem-solvers who often expect the same qualities from their teachers
- As "digital immigrants," are proficient with technology and adaptable to new advances but recall a time when technology was not as prevalent (Borges et al., 2006; Borges et al., 2010)

MILLENNIALS (BORN 1981–1995)

- Are highly accomplished
- Are collaborative and accustomed to working in teams
- Appreciate rules and structure, including individualized teaching and learning
- Don't just value, but expect feedback and praise, which contributes to the perception that they are entitled (the "everyone-gets-a-trophy generation")
- Tend to be risk-averse
- Are optimistic as a group, having lived through the New York City terrorist attack of 9/11, seen the rise of technology, and experienced great change
- As "digital pioneers," view technology as a necessity (Eckleberry-Hunt & Tucciarone, 2011; Desy et al., 2017; Twenge, 2009)

GEN Z (BORN 1996–2015)

- More racially and ethnically diverse than previous cohorts
- More well-educated than their predecessors

- As "digital natives," do not know a world without technology
- Prefer face-to-face to digital interactions in the workplace
- Face mental health challenges:
  - They are more prone to psychological distress than earlier generations
  - Their dependence on technology is correlated with greater levels of depression, anxiety, and isolation
- Possess a strong sense of social responsibility
- Value mentorship and collaboration—but also quiet, independent work (Plochocki, 2019; Chunta et al., 2021, DiMattio & Hudacek, 2020; Schenarts, 2019; Seibert, 2021)

After the workshop, Dr. Forss has a chance to orient herself to the characteristics of various generational cohorts. This has opened her eyes to the different lenses through which her learners may view the world, based on their common lived experiences. She has found this very helpful, but she worries that these different viewpoints may cause challenges or tensions in the workplace.

Common Tension Points

The following are common tension points specific to intergenerational work environments, such as the labour floor, that have been described in the literature on this topic (Myers & Sadaghiani, 2010; Borges et al., 2010; Murnaghan et al., 2011):

1. Engaging with technology
2. Expectations for providing feedback
3. Navigating autonomy and support

ENGAGING WITH TECHNOLOGY

Example:

You are doing a small group teaching session on methods for inducing labour. One of the Millennial learners is looking at their phone the entire time. You are unsure whether this learner is checking social media or texting a friend, or if they are engaged in something related to the topic, such as looking up resources or pulling up the latest trial data. You contemplate asking the learner, right then and there, about being on the phone. You decide not to, and end up leaving the session feeling irritated, with the perception that the learner is uninterested and even disrespectful—but wondering, "Is it them or is it me?"

Potential Tension Points

- Millennials are digital pioneers and Gen Z are digital natives, while Boomers and Gen Xers are digital immigrants
- Different generations adopt and use technology in different ways, including . . .
    - How we interact with the technology in our daily work and lives
    - What we think is acceptable and desirable—i.e., what kinds of technology use one appreciates or accepts versus what one deems rude or a sign of disengagement
- Instant or near-instant messaging capacity via email, text, or social media has changed our expectations around the immediacy of communication

While changes in the use of technology can facilitate real-time remote interaction and rapid responses to urgent questions, it can also cause blurring of personal and professional boundaries.

EXPECTATIONS FOR PROVIDING FEEDBACK

Example:

You fill out an end-of-rotation evaluation on a Gen Z learner whose skills are below those of their peers—and your expectations. You had provided some tips to the learner throughout the rotation verbally, including how to properly perform a cervical exam and where to find additional learning resources. You also spent a fair amount of time teaching the learner how to tie a hand knot. However, when the learner receives the final rotation feedback, they become quite agitated and report that they never received any negative feedback throughout the rotation, so feel this final evaluation is unfair.

Potential Tension Points

- Boomers and Gen Xers are accustomed to most formal feedback being delivered at defined points (e.g., as mid- or end-rotation evaluations), and often rely on their own self-assessment in between evaluations
- Millennials report a higher desire for a steady stream of feedback on a regular basis. This is significantly more resource-intensive, which can create a mismatch between learner expectations and what the teacher can realistically provide
- Some may perceive a learner's desire for a constant stream of positive and reassuring feedback as being resistant to constructive feedback

NAVIGATING AUTONOMY AND SUPPORT

Example:

You are accustomed to working independently and recall being expected to do so as a learner (It was a point of pride for you that during your training, you rarely woke staff up to ask them a question overnight). You feel that you learned by taking on responsibility early in your training. You like to give learners the same opportunity to develop their skills. You notice, however, that often the Millennial learners with whom you are working seek you out for support early in management and require a lot of hand-holding.

Potential Tension Points

- Millennial learners are more risk-averse than older generations
- While Boomers and Gen Xers were trained in an environment with the adage "see one, do one, teach one," this no longer applies, and is viewed as unnecessary risk-taking
- Teamwork and collaboration are strengths for Millennials. A potential tension arises when learners expect this collaborative style from teachers, which differs from the independent, self-directed learning style to which their Gen X and Boomer teachers may be accustomed.
- Millennial learners' desire for support may be viewed as neediness or lack of self-direction

- Teachers' desire to provide opportunities for independence may in fact leave the Millennial learner feeling unsafe or unsupported

Integration and Strategies

Once familiar with generational cohorts, challenges, and tension points, you might use the following strategies to address them (Roberts et al., 2012):

1. Orient yourself and your learner
2. Identify the core values of the profession
3. Facilitate critical thinking
4. Communicate with clarity
5. Connect with learners
6. Engage technology wisely

ORIENT YOURSELF AND YOUR LEARNER

The first step in overcoming intergenerational barriers to learning is for teachers to orient themselves to their learners. It is particularly important in intergenerational settings for teachers to identify . . .

- The characteristics of their cohorts
- The generational values or societal influences at play in the learning environment
- How learning might be impacted by these factors

The second step is to orient Millennials to the expectations of Gen X and Boomer teachers, as well as to the expectations of the profession in general. This two-way orientation can help facilitate a mutual understanding between the teacher and learner.

Labour and delivery environments are not always easy for newcomers to navigate. There is often an established hierarchy and unwritten expectations and norms. This may be particularly challenging for Millennials, who relish learning in teams that are less hierarchical. Some techniques that may help the learner's experience in labour and delivery are . . .

- Introducing learners to the nursing and obstetrical staff as junior colleagues
- Orienting learners to what is expected of them on the rotation and the culture of the labour and delivery environment

Example:

You are working with a new Gen Z learner in clinic. You take time to ask where they are from and what their previous experience with prenatal patients is. They explain that most of their clerkship training was in a busy, high-risk obstetrical office, where they tended to occupy an observational role, never being expected to manage patient care. You explain that as a learner in your clinic, expectations are different, and that they are primarily managing rather than observing care. However, you make it clear that you are available for support as needed. You discuss the learner's comfort level with the equipment used during a prenatal visit.

IDENTIFY CORE VALUES OF THE PROFESSION

In addition to orienting learners to the environment and culture of the labour floor, perinatal care teachers can highlight what they do that is different and unique. Learners will interact with and be taught by many health professionals involved in caring for patients throughout pregnancy and birth. However, it is only by working with professional role models that they will fully come to understand the core values of the profession they are joining. As Millennials highly value meaning to their work, explaining *why* we do what we do may help them connect with their educators and their own clinical work.

Example:

One night on call, you and your Millennial resident are enjoying a late dinner after a day filled with deliveries. Your resident asks why you decided to go into family medicine and not obstetrics if you love delivering babies so much. You explain that you chose family medicine because you felt it was where your values best aligned: caring for patients throughout the life cycle, with the opportunity to work with multigenerational families and provide comprehensive care—that includes perinatal care. As a family physician who provides intrapartum perinatal care, you are able to demonstrate advanced clinical skills, an approach to birth as a natural event, and care for the mother-baby dyad into the future.

Helping Millennials familiarize themselves with their teacher's values connects them and orients them to the core values of their chosen profession. This sense of inclusion in the community of practice is essential to a positive learning environment.

FACILITATE CRITICAL THINKING

The role of the teacher is to facilitate, curate, and interpret knowledge, rather than to simply provide it in a traditional, didactic manner. In the current digital environment, learners can instantly look up the answers to questions. The role of the teacher is to assist in the *understanding* and *application* of this knowledge.

Teachers can facilitate critical thinking by encouraging learners to develop to their full potential by analyzing their performances, instructing them in relevant skills and providing encouragement rather than solely imparting information and knowledge. The metaphor of "teacher as coach" works well, where the teacher offers mentorship and support through feedback on performance and paying attention to a learner's strengths and weaknesses.

Example:

You are supervising a 3rd-year Gen Z medical student while running a prenatal/ newborn clinic. Your student wishes to discuss the management of two babies that presented with jaundice. In one case, you sent the baby in for a repeat bilirubin, and in the other, you sent the baby home. Your student is curious as to why different management plans were used. Rather than doing a didactic teaching session on managing hyperbilirubinemia, you say:

"Review the Canadian Pediatric Society's hyperbilirubinemia guidelines. We can discuss them further tomorrow and address any questions you have. Also, take a minute to download the Bili-Tool app. Finally, let's just chat about some reassuring and worrisome features to look for."

In this way, the learner can do the book-learning on their own time. The teacher can use their clinical experience to augment the learner's understanding by discussing application of the knowledge in a variety of different circumstances. The goal is to stimulate learning and facilitate the development of adaptive expertise. This involves the teacher asking the learner probing questions rather than just providing answers (see Chapter 3).

COMMUNICATE WITH CLARITY

Intergenerational communication should be particularly clear and straightforward to avoid misunderstanding. To accomplish this, you should . . .

- Identify the competencies expected of learners and communicate them distinctly to them
- Tailor learning plans specific to Millennial needs
- Provide specific feedback that is fair, transparent, frequent, and in real time
- Support feedback with specific examples so that it fully resonates

Example:

You are working with a 1st-year Millennial resident on call for the first time and anticipate that you will be asked to evaluate them. You are intentional about giving the resident specific and tailored feedback to help her improve and to be deliberate about labelling it as feedback.

You address the resident: "Just so we're on the same page, let's review the expected competencies. Maybe we can pick a couple that we really want to focus on during our shift together and try to address them. At the end of the shift, I'll be filling out an evaluation for you so we can review some of your strengths and identify some areas you may still need some work on. Do you have any questions before we get started?"

At the end of the shift, you sit down with the resident and say: "I'd like to give you some feedback based on what I observed during your shift. I thought you did a great job with communicating with the patient. You were very diligent in explaining our assessment and plan with her and ensuring she understood and agreed with the plan. Something I think you still need some work on is your cervical assessments. You seemed unsure of your exams and your assessment was often discrepant from mine. Why do you think that was? How comfortable are you with your cervical exams?"

You then provide some coaching for the resident: "Let's come up with an action plan to help you develop this skill a bit. There is a great photo online that shows different items and their diameter, which can help to visualize things—for example, a penny is 2 centimetres, an Oreo cookie is 4 centimetres, a pop can is 6 centimetres, and so on. It's worth looking up."

Clear and intentional communication is essential in interacting with Millennials—especially with respect to expectations and assessments. The key is transparent communication and a coaching style of teaching where specific strategies for improvement are provided.

CONNECT WITH LEARNERS

Building connections both with and amongst learners is essential for teachers. There are a variety of ways to do this while working together on the labour and delivery floor. In fact, spending time together on call is one of the best opportunities teachers have to gain insight into a learner's work habits, cognitive and procedural skills, and attitudes. It also represents an excellent opportunity to build the teacher-learner relationship in the manner sought after by Millennials. While Gen Xers are accustomed to independence and pride themselves on not bothering the teacher, Millennials tend to appreciate or expect the personal connection and close supervision.

You can connect with the learner at the start of the shift (or even prior to the shift) by . . .

- Discussing how you will communicate while on call
- Gauging the learner's prior experience and comfort level with the tasks that will be expected of them
- Inquiring about the learner's personal goals and what gaps they are trying to fill

Taking the time to have these conversations ahead of a busy shift allows the teacher to better discern what level of responsibility may be appropriate for a learner and where they may wish to have growth opportunities.

To further develop the teacher-learner relationship, you might try to . . .

- Flatten traditional hierarchies
- Make yourself more accessible outside of your in-person time together via email or text (though this may present new challenges, like the blurring of distinctions between professional and personal time and space)

Example:

When on call, you look ahead at the schedule and plan to connect with the resident before handover. You take the opportunity to introduce yourself and find out about the learner's experiences and interests and to discuss if they have any learning goals for the shift. You also let them know you are available to answer any questions—or if they need anything else.

On shift, you have some downtime between cervical checks. You say: "I know you're new to the city—how are you settling in? What challenges are you finding with the transition to residency and specifically around your perinatal care rotation? Would it be helpful for me to sit with you and answer your questions or help troubleshoot any issues you have?"

One of the advantages of long on-call shifts is that there is often downtime, which affords us the luxury of sitting together for periods of time and getting to know each other. Millennials value these personal connections more than earlier generations typically have. They appreciate knowing that their teachers are interested both in their learning and in them as people. It is important for teachers to demonstrate that they are invested in the success of their learners.

ENGAGE TECHNOLOGY WISELY

Think back to the tension points described in our section on "Engaging with Technology."

Example:

After some consideration, you reflect on the fact that while you would never check a phone while a teacher is talking, your learners may have a more integrated view of technology, regarding their devices as extensions of their thoughts and learning processes. You decide that the next time you are leading a small group, you will . . .

- *Set expectations ahead of time regarding the use of personal devices during the session to ensure everyone is on the same page*
- *Try integrating an interactive activity into the session where the learners might use their device for a specific purpose (e.g., texting a response or creating a word cloud)*
- *Ask learners for their input regarding which online or point-of-care tools they access via their devices—and what they do or do not find helpful*

While virtual learning has been a component of education for the better part of the 2000s, COVID–19—and the lockdowns and physical distancing associated with it—has elevated technology and online learning to an essential part of teaching. This has pushed Boomer and Gen X teachers to quickly adopt these new techniques, which their Millennial and Gen Z learners—digital pioneers and natives—are equipped to adopt.

Teachers should consider the following:

- Using blogs, podcasts, webinars, asynchronous lectures (where a learner watches a previously recorded session on their own time), games, online modules, or interactive activities
- Recognizing that effective e-learning tools are interactive and engaging, technologically advanced, and aesthetically appealing—and facilitate connections between teachers and learners
- Recognizing that the method of digital communication itself can send a message (e.g., email, being asynchronous, contributes to the formality of communication, while text messaging has expectations of immediacy and informality attached)
- The need to use technology wisely and deliberately—not just because it is expected

Example:

You are working with an experienced resident whose core skills are very good. However, it is clear they are not yet comfortable with perineal suturing. They ask you for a good resource they can review on their own. You do all of the following:

- *Refer them to a cherished perinatal textbook (it is a classic that is now online)*
- *Recall a great article you once read and email it to them*
- *Text/email/WhatsApp/Airdrop them an instructional video*

The essential message is that good teaching is enhanced with—not replaced by—technology.

Conclusion

The majority of our discussion has been focused on Millennial learners and their tensions with their Boomer and Gen X teachers. It is important to recognize that Millennial learners are a diverse group and that we need to be conscious of stereotyping. A caveat to all this advice is that evidence that adaptations in teaching styles in response to generational characteristics result in more competent learners is yet to be published.

In addition, many Millennials are early career teachers, and those who are part of Gen Z are becoming the next cohort of learners, with their own characteristics and challenges. Teachers should have flexible styles and the ability to adapt to the changing needs of learners, while maintaining the core values that are central to the practice of perinatal care in their discipline.

REFERENCES

Aaron, M., & Levenberg, P. (2014). The millennials in medicine: Tips for teaching the next generation of physicians. Journal of Academic Ophthalmology, 7, e017-e020. http://dx.doi.org/ 10.1055/s-0034-1396088.

Adams, D. (2002). The salmon of doubt: Hitchhiking the galaxy one last time. Harmony.

Borges, N.J., Manuel, R.S., Elam, C.L., & Jones, B.J. (2010). Differences in motives between millennial and generation X medical students. Medical Education, 44, 570-576. doi:10.1111/j.1365-2923.2010.03633.x.

Borges, N.J., Manuel, R.S., Elam, C.L., & Jones, B.J. (2006). Comparing millennial and generation X medical students at one medical school. Academic Medicine, 81, 571-576. doi: 10.1097/01.acm.0000225222.38078.47

Chunta, K., Shellenbarger, T., & Chicca, J. (2021). Generation Z students in the online environment: Strategies for nurse educators. Nurse Educator, 46, 87-91. doi: 10.1097/NNE.0000000000000872.

Desy, J.R., Reed, D.A., & Wolansky, A.P. (2017). Milestones and millennials: A perfect pairing - competency-based medical education and the learning preferences of generation Y. Mayo Clinic Proceedings, 92, 243-250. doi: 10.1016/j.mayocp.2016.10.026

DiMattio, M.J.K., & Hudacek, S.S. (2020). Educating generation Z: Psychosocial dimensions of the clinical learning environment that predict student satisfaction. Nurse Education in Practice, 49, 102901. doi: 10.1016/j.nepr.2020.102901

Eckleberry-Hunt, J., & Tucciarone, J. (2011). The challenges and opportunities of teaching "generation Y." Journal of Graduate Medical Education, 3, 458-461. doi: 10.4300/JGME-03-04-15

Murnaghan, M.L, Forte, M., Choy, I.C., & Abner, E. (2011). Innovations in Teaching and Learning in the Clinical Setting for Postgraduate Medical Education. Members of the FMEC PG consortium, 12-13. https://pdfslide.net/documents/16-innovations-in-teaching-and-learning-in-the-clinical-16-innovations-in.html

Myers, K.K., & Sadaghiani, K. (2010). Millennials in the Workplace: A Communication Perspective on Millennials' Organizational Relationships and Performance. Journal of Business Psychology, 25(2), 225-38.

Plochocki, J.H. (2019). Several ways generation Z may shape the medical school landscape. Journal of Medical Education and Curricular Development, 6, 1-4. https://doi.org/10.1177/2382120519884325

Roberts, D.H., Newman, L.R., & Schwartzstein, R.M. (2012). Twelve tips for facilitating millennials' learning. Medical Teacher, 34, 274-278. doi: 10.3109/0142159X.2011.613498

Schenarts, P.J. (2020). Now arriving: Surgical trainees from generation Z. Journal of Surgical Education, 77, 246-253. doi: 10.1016/j.jsurg.2019.09.004

Seibert, S.A. (2021). Problem-based learning; A strategy to foster generation Z's critical thinking and perseverance. Teaching and Learning in Nursing, 16, 85-88. doi: 10.1016/j.teln.2020.09.002

Twenge, J.M. (2009). Generational changes and their impact in the classroom: teaching generation me. Medical Education, 43, 389-405. doi: 10.1111/j.1365-2923.2009.03310.x

Williams, V.N., Medina, J., Medina, A., & Clifton, S. (2017). Bridging the millennial generation expectation gap: Perspectives and strategies for physician and interprofessional faculty. The American Journal of the Medical Sciences, 353, 109-115. https://doi.org/10.1016/j.amjms.2016.12.004

Chapter 7

MENTORSHIP IN PERINATAL CARE

David Eisen, David White

Dr. George Cochrane has been assigned to oversee the onboarding of a recent family medicine graduate who has been recruited by his hospital and has applied for perinatal care privileges. Dr. Cochrane realizes the process has become more formal since he joined the hospital and seeks to learn more about it. He would like to make the process more welcoming, supportive, and nurturing, while ensuring it upholds high standards of care and the hospital's requirements. He attends a workshop at his local university to learn more about mentorship.

Introduction

Mentorship has long been recognized as key to successful development in virtually every human endeavour (Kammeyer-Mueller & Judge, 2008). This chapter begins with an overview of basic mentorship concepts and then provides practical tips relevant to family doctors who practise perinatal care.

A mentor is defined as "a person who acts as guide and adviser to another person, especially one who is younger and less experienced; more generally: a person who offers support and guidance to another" (Simpson & Weiner, 1989). The term originates in Greek mythology, in which Odysseus asks his old friend Mentor to advise and educate his young son Telemachus while Odysseus is away fighting in the Trojan war (Homer & Mackail, 1903).[1]

---

1   Homer's "Odyssey" portrays Mentor as elderly and ineffectual. Fortunately for Telemachus, Athena, the goddess of wisdom, occasionally disguises herself as Mentor to provide guidance.

The concept of mentoring has evolved considerably from its origins. Mentorship relationships come in many forms, along a continuum from informal, short-term relationships to formal, long-term ones (Berk et al., 2005). Mentoring relationships should be voluntary and initiated by the mentee, though there are many examples of programs with assigned mentors or mentorships developing from the identification of a mentee (or protégé) by an experienced practitioner. A mentorship is . . .

- A helping relationship focused on achievement
- A relationship that consists of emotional and psychological support, direct assistance with professional development, and role-modelling
- A reciprocal relationship, where both mentor and mentee derive emotional or tangible benefits
- A personal relationship that involves direct interaction
- A relationship that emphasizes the mentor's greater experience, influence, and achievement in a particular organization (Jacobi, 1991)

Why Mentorship?

Example:

You have always admired your family medicine preceptor, who provides perinatal care. Having just obtained hospital privileges as you start your own career as a family physician providing perinatal care, you aspire to be just like her: a dedicated, skilled clinician who makes a point of attending as many of her patients' births as possible. However, with two young children in your two-career family, you are uncertain how to manage the needs of family and the demands of practice. You want to connect with potential mentors in your setting who could provide advice, support, and role-modelling of how to manage practice, family commitments, and personal well-being. To prepare yourself for seeking out a mentor, you explore the qualities and characteristics that contribute to effective mentoring.

Physicians recognize that mentorship is important and correlates with professional success (Straus & Sackett, 2014). Successful mentoring requires . . .

- Commitment and interpersonal skills on the part of the mentor and mentee
- A facilitating environment (Sambunjak et al., 2010)

Family physicians value receiving mentorship for their overall career, clinical practice, teaching, leadership, and work-life balance (Stubbs et al., 2016). This may be particularly relevant for perinatal care, where work-life balance can be a particular challenge. Supportive teachers and positive role models influence family medicine residents' decisions to include obstetrics in their practice (Koppula et al., 2012), and effective mentors are often role models as well (Biringer et al., 2018). Mentorship has been recommended as a strategy for preventing burnout among midwives (Jordan et al., 2013) and family physicians who provide perinatal care (Goldstein et al., 2018). Mentorship is an important strategy for supporting recent graduates from family medicine programs who want to incorporate perinatal care into their practice (Koppula et al., 2014).

The benefit to a mentee is widely recognized as the purpose of the mentoring relationship. Organizations are also beneficiaries of mentoring, however, experiencing outcomes that include enhanced communication, reduced turnover, and greater commitment (Baugh & Fagenson-Eland, 2008). That the mentor benefits from the interaction is also evident, though this is less widely recognized. Mentors themselves experience invigoration of their interest in their discipline, along with a sense of personal and professional growth. Mentors take satisfaction in helping mentees address the problems they face. They enjoy "giving back" and witnessing their mentees develop. Mentorship also brings challenges, as in any human relationship or undertaking (Straus & Sackett, 2014). Mentorship problems are outlined later in the chapter, along with recommendations for how to recognize and address them.

The Mentor

Example:

You have been teaching medical students and including them in your family medicine perinatal care practice for several years when one of the students asks if you would continue as his mentor after the rotation ends. You are 5 years into practice and feel uncertain about being a mentor. For advice, you turn to a colleague, who was your own mentor when you were a resident. You reflect on your experience with him. He did not try to influence you to include perinatal care in your practice but shared what it meant to him personally. Those honest conversations had a powerful impact on you. You realize that you could bring the same quality to your relationship with your mentee.

TYPES OF MENTORSHIP

"The mentor" has evolved over time and now takes many forms beyond the senior, respected elder. Mentorship as both concept and practice has a relationship to activities like teaching, role-modelling, and coaching. Describing these varied forms and related activities will help us develop a deeper understanding of how to engage in and support mentorships.

Traditional Mentoring

"Traditional" mentoring is based on Homer's classical description of the relationship between Mentor and Odysseus's son Telemachus—an elder guiding and supporting the development of a young protégé.[2] In medicine, it is framed as

> A process whereby an experienced, highly regarded, empathetic person (the mentor) guides another (usually younger) individual (the mentee) in the development and re-examination of their own ideas, learning, and personal and professional development. The mentor, who often (but not necessarily) works in the same organization or field as the mentee, achieves this by listening or talking in confidence to the mentee. (SCOPUS, 1998)

Mentoring relationships may be assigned as part of formal programs, such as those that exist in many medical schools and residencies (Frei et al., 2010). Such mentoring programs are becoming more common for new faculty of medical schools. Or, mentorship relationships may just evolve spontaneously between colleagues who work in similar fields or settings.

---

2   "Mentor" entered the English language as a capitalized word in direct reference to the character in Greek mythology.

Peer Mentoring

Peer mentoring differs from conventional mentorship in that the relationship is one of equality between members of the peer group (Holbeche, 1996). This is useful in "flat" organizations where there are relatively few senior advisers. Its key characteristic is mutuality: it combines peer support with guidance that reflects shared experience (McManus & Russell, 2008). Hearing about a peer's challenges that are similar to your own not only provides you an opportunity to assist them, but also gives perspective on your own issues.

Mentorship Groups

Mentorship groups may occur when a mentor gets together with several mentees who are in similar organizations or career stages. It can also be an aspect of peer mentoring (P-Sontag et al., 2008). Mentorship groups can evolve out of teacher-student relationships. Another form of mentorship groups can come out of an individual identifying a number of people who are part of a supportive constellation or "developmental network" (McManus & Russel, 2008). Some members of the network may be traditional mentors, while others may be family members, supervisors, peers, co-workers, and friends. This network exists for the individual who forms the relationships but does not meet together as a formal entity. These models are generally informal, developing from the mentee's own initiative but can also be part of formal programs that carefully match mentors and mentees (P-Sontag et al., 2008). The development of peer mentoring has been identified as a characteristic of supportive obstetrical care groups of family physicians (Koppula et al., 2011). "Practice mentoring" has potential to encourage recent family medicine graduates who express concerns about lifestyle to include or continue to include perinatal care in their practice (Barreto et al., 2019).

Coaching, Role-Modelling, and Teaching

The word "mentor" is sometimes used interchangeably with "coach" or "role model." It is better to distinguish between these concepts and retain clarity in the use of these terms (Straus & Sackett, 2014). Coaching and mentorship share some characteristics and diverge in other ways (Marcdante & Simpson, 2018). Coaches observe players, performers, or teams and provide specific feedback to support deliberate practice of tasks or skills (Ericsson, 2008). Mentors do not necessarily directly observe their mentees, but in hearing about a setback or stumbling block, may provide advice on strategies to improve their outcome. A mentor's responsibilities also go far beyond this, including providing emotional support, opening doors of opportunity for the mentee, and helping them explore the meaning and significance of their experiences. Coaches occasionally do this for select individuals (thus becoming mentors), but it is not part of everyday coaching.

A role model sets an example, providing a learning opportunity for the observer. A mentor is often a role model for many colleagues, but this does not entail the emotional investment and personal interaction that characterizes their relationship with a mentee.

Clinical teachers generally aspire to be positive role models for their trainees. Teaching perinatal care commonly involves coaching—especially with regards to procedural skills. Teacher-trainee relationships that continue throughout residency may incorporate some attributes of mentorship but are limited in scope and constrained by the supervisory and evaluation components. Some of these relationships evolve into ongoing mentorships that extend beyond graduation. An example will be described later in the chapter.

THE MENTOR: QUALITIES AND BEST PRACTICES

The qualities of effective mentors can be described in three categories: personal attributes, behaviours toward mentees, and professional stature (Straus & Sackett, 2014; Williams et al., 2004).

Personal Attributes

Effective mentors are . . .

- Enthusiastic
- Understanding
- Non-judgmental
- Patient
- Trustworthy
- Motivating
- Self-appraising

Behaviours

Productive approaches for interacting with mentees are . . .

- Active listening
- Being accessible
- Supporting their best interests
- Identifying their potential strengths
- Assisting them in defining and reaching their goals
- Holding a high standard for their achievements
- Trying to be compatible with their practice style, vision, and personality

Professional Stature

The mentor's professional stature in the traditional model is based on . . .

- Their level of success in their field
- The level of respect they command from their colleagues
- Their connections to sources of additional help
- Their power or authority within a particular professional organization or work setting

Mentors may have these attributes and engage in these behaviours to varying degrees, but all will play a role in their mentoring. These elements are also at play in less traditional mentoring relationships like peer mentoring and mentorship groups. Although participants in these types of mentoring relationships may lack significant power in their setting, they usually connect and form groups with others who have attained respect, success, and connections commensurate with their career stage or station within an organization.

Power and authority allow a mentor to open doors and facilitate networks for their mentee. They are also crucial in circumstances when a mentee needs protection. An example might be their ability to stand up for a mentee who is bullied, subjected to unduly harsh criticism for an error or misstep, or excluded from or passed over for advancement. These situations are common in health-care organizations, frequently affecting women and under-represented minorities (Coombs & King, 2005; Fnais et al., 2014; Pololi et al., 2013).

The Mentee

Example:

You make a mid-career move to a teaching hospital, where you continue practising perinatal care. The chief of obstetrics and gynecology at the hospital is an experienced and highly respected specialist. Shortly after your arrival, he invites you to his office, asking for advice about a personnel issue in labour and delivery. He indicates that he is seeking a fresh perspective from someone with experience at a different institution. You are flattered that a senior and more knowledgeable colleague would request your opinion, and you respond as best you can. The chief listens intently and tells you that he finds your advice helpful. After further invitations to provide feedback to the chief, you come to the realization that these meetings are his way of mentoring and introducing you to the culture and structure—both formal and informal—of perinatal care at the hospital. The relationship continues for many years, and you are deeply grateful for it. You never ask him why he chose you, but you work hard to be a good mentee.

CHARACTERISTICS OF A SUCCESSFUL MENTEE

Successful mentees are . . .

- Proactive
- Willing to learn
- Selective in accepting advice from their mentors
- Committed
- Passionate about succeeding in their careers
- Self-reflective
- Willing to reveal their flaws to their mentors

The mentee-mentor relationship is more productive when mentees . . .

- Initiate the relationship
- Prepare for meetings with their mentor
- Provide an outline of their activities
- Complete agreed-upon tasks
- Respond to feedback (Williams et al., 2004; Sambunjak et al., 2010)

Not every successful mentee requires all these characteristics or needs to perform all these tasks. For example, the scenario that introduced this section described a mentor who initiated a relationship with a newcomer at his hospital. Nevertheless, its success depends on initiative and commitment from both of them.

Finding a Mentor

There are two broad categories under which mentoring relationships arise: formal and informal. Informal mentorship can evolve from . . .

- Clinical interactions between more experienced and less experienced colleagues
- Teacher-student relationships
- Employer-employee relationships
- Supervisor-subordinate or trainer-trainee relationships

In informal relationships, senior colleagues may be unaware that some of those with whom they regularly interact regard them as mentors (Stubbs et al., 2016).

Some organizations establish formal mentorship programs using a variety of support mechanisms, which may include . . .

- Assigning mentor-mentee dyads
- Facilitating mentees in identifying potential mentors
- Setting mentorship as an expectation where successful mentees take the initiative via strategies like asking peers or senior colleagues for suggestions, setting up preliminary meetings with potential mentors, and formally interviewing their top choices to formalize expectations and commitment
- Outlining expectations for mentors and mentees (e.g., frequency of meetings)
- Providing training for mentors
- Appointing a director for the mentorship program who has the responsibility of assessing and improving its effectiveness (Straus, & Sackett, 2014)

The Mentoring Relationship

Effective mentoring relationships are characterized by . . .

- A personal connection
- A set of shared values around how one approaches research, clinical work, and social life
- Mutual respect for each other's time, effort, and expectations
- Clear expectations
- Reciprocity in efforts and rewards (Straus & Sackett, 2014)

The role of gender and ethnicity in mentoring relationships is attracting prominent attention. Physicians who are women and/or part of a minority group are more likely to agree that gender and ethnicity are important, whereas men perceive that it makes little difference (Williams et al., 2004). Female family doctors practising perinatal care found that the women had mentors but missed having role models (Carroll et al., 1995). Trainees in family medicine express various views regarding having a mentor of the same gender or similar age but are consistent regarding the importance of the personal mentor attributes described earlier in the chapter (Belle Brown et al., 2012). Graduates of family medicine programs who incorporate perinatal care into their practices appear to have integrated the attitudes of their mentors, believing that delivering babies is not disruptive to personal life (Godwin et al., 2002).

Connecting regularly is essential for effective mentoring. Some formal mentorship programs mandate a minimum number or frequency of scheduled meetings, but this is not a requirement for success. Many fruitful mentorship relationships thrive on the basis of ad hoc meetings, informal occasions such as coffees or lunches, or working on a shared project. That said, health professionals are notoriously busy and need to book ahead for time together.

In addition to the characteristics described above, formal mentorship programs commonly provide supports, such as reminders to meet, possible topics to discuss, and tips for both mentors and mentees. Formal mentoring relationships have evolved to include the various models discussed above, such as peer mentorship, team mentoring, mentoring circles, and structured networks. Formal mentoring programs claim to have numerous advantages for both mentees and organizations, including creating a culture of supportive relationships and introducing new recruits to the organization's values, structure, and informal mechanisms. Formal mentorship programs have been used to support diversity, but they have been described as "the poor cousin" to informal mentoring, with the latter contributing to mentees experiencing a greater sense of support and career success (Baugh & Fagenson-Eland, 2008). In formal programs, care in matching mentees and mentors contributes to success (P-Sontag et al., 2008). Formal mentorships are commonly time-limited, but some continue as informal relationships after the assignment ends.

Challenges

We have looked at how things should work in an ideal world. However, as in every human undertaking, elements of mentorships can and do go wrong. Prevention is ideal, but recognizing and intervening are necessary when the relationship is going off the rails. Key challenges include . . .

- Lack of time
- Lack of commitment
- Failing to schedule meetings
- Late cancellations or no-shows
- A mentee failing to complete agreed-upon tasks
- A mentee not responding to feedback

In teaching settings, there are barriers that result in problems, such as . . .

- Fewer than 50% of medical students having a mentor
- In certain fields, fewer than 20% of faculty members having a mentor
- Women perceiving that they have more difficulty finding mentors than men (Sambunjak et al., 2006)

As an example, family doctors who are dedicated to engaging in mentorship relationships face the constraints of limited time and competing demands. Challenges specific to mentoring in perinatal care include . . .

- The demanding nature of practice
- Inherent conflicts in striking work-life balance given desire to provide continuity of care and the importance of 24/7 coverage
- Institutional requirements

- Hierarchy in labour and delivery settings
- The highly variable nature of the labouring and birth process
- The wide range of individual patient needs and preferences (Quaas et al., 2009; Tracy et al., 2004)

Mentors are—by definition—those who are experienced in their field. The extraordinary variability of preferences and approaches to birth among all involved, from the pregnant person to their supporters and caregivers, means a mentor's advice—based on their own experiences, perceptions, and preferences—may not be relevant or applicable to the needs of the mentee. Mentees may address this issue by having multiple mentors (Brown et al., 2012).

There is a power differential in the mentor-mentee relationship, and this can be abused if the mentee's goals are subverted to serve those of the mentor. Inappropriate behaviour may involve bullying or sexual harassment. Institutional policies and practices, such as having an individual responsible for supervising the mentorship, may assist in preventing issues—or addressing them if they arise. This supervisor could be a director of a formal mentorship program or the department chief (Sambunjak et al., 2010). Rigid hierarchies—formerly common in perinatal care settings—increase the risk of these types of inappropriate behaviours. Organizational cultures that promote teamwork, interprofessional cooperation, and respect for all care providers help create an environment in which healthy mentoring relationships can thrive.

Sometimes a mentor-mentee relationship evolves into a supportive, non-exploitative, enduring friendship—or even a romantic relationship. This significant qualitative change necessitates ending the mentoring. The couple may recognize this and arrange for another mentor to take over the mentee. If not, their friends or senior colleagues should intervene to facilitate a transition (Straus & Sackett, 2014).

Key Opportunities for Mentorship: Practical examples

DIFFICULT CASE, BAD OUTCOME

Example:

Your long-time mentee approaches you after a very difficult case in labour and delivery, which resulted in an imperfect outcome and a patient complaint. As you listen to the story, you realize that the patient's complaint has merit. This is a stressor on the mentor-mentee relationship: you are supportive of your mentee's work, but not the care of this particular patient. You explain your concerns and reservations frankly. You share your opinion on what might have been done differently, acknowledging that hindsight is always 20/20. As you talk, your mentee acknowledges that she would have preferred whole-hearted support. Nevertheless, you both realize that honest, constructive feedback is the foundation of the mentor-mentee relationship.

Challenges abound in perinatal care, and bad outcomes will occur despite our best efforts. This scenario illustrates that a robust mentorship is built on a foundation of trust and honest feedback. Critical to mentoring in this situation is that the mentor expresses support for the mentee while critiquing her role in the specific situation. In a supportive environment, the mentee is able to acknowledge their shortcomings, share their feelings honestly, and absorb the lessons of the experience.

BECOMING A MENTOR TO A COLLEAGUE

The scenario that opens the chapter describes Dr. Cochrane, an experienced family physician who would like to transform his hospital's perinatal care onboarding process from a supervisory relationship to a nurturing, supportive one. In recognizing this, he takes an important first step on the path to becoming an effective mentor. The principles of good mentorship then come into focus: personal connection, shared values, mutual respect, clear expectations, and reciprocal efforts and benefits.

As a mentor to this new grad, Dr. Cochrane can respect their skills and up-to-date training while using his depth of experience and institutional familiarity for the mentorship role. He can set clear expectations in terms of clinical skills expected at the new grad's level of career, as well as the values and culture of the perinatal care providers at the hospital. Finally, he can acknowledge that they are both on the same path—just at different points along the way. They will soon be sharing calls and patients and taking care of each other's clinical, teaching, research, and other responsibilities.

Working together as colleagues places mentor and mentee on more even ground, minimizing power differentials (Jackson et al., 2003). Supportive supervision and mentorship can build confidence in perinatal care skills, which is often lacking in recent graduates (Biringer et al., 2019).

Context and institutional culture are crucial in creating conditions in which a mentorship can thrive. The senior leaders in a healthcare organization set the tone and expectations for behaviour. This goes beyond statements of mission, vision, and values to how those aspirations are lived every day throughout the organization.

CHANGES TO A MENTORSHIP AS MENTOR AND MENTEE'S CAREERS PROGRESS

Example:

Early in your career, you worked closely with a senior colleague as your mentor. He was particularly supportive when you first joined the hospital as a perinatal care provider and was very proud when you were appointed chief of family medicine obstetrics. Lately, the delivery room nurses have been noticing that he appears nervous and lacking in confidence when he is on call and providing care for patients of his colleagues. They report their concerns to you, given your role as chief, responsible for family medicine perinatal care privileges. The nurses frankly question his competence. You feel awkward about this, given your past relationship as his mentee. But, you want to support your colleague and call group partner while carrying out your duty to ensure safe care by competent practitioners. When you meet with him, he tells you that he is approaching the point of retirement. He indicates that two of his own patients are due in the following 3 months, and he wants to attend their births before relinquishing obstetric privileges.

Changes in a mentorship can range from smooth to heart wrenching. In most cases, the evolution is situational and understood implicitly by both parties. Institutional mentorships may endure after one member of the mentorship dyad moves away, but they commonly fade or end. As described earlier in the chapter, the relationship may evolve into a friendship, or to intermittent, long-distance mentoring. In the scenario we illustrated to open this section, the mentee has progressed to a stage of respect, responsibility, and power within the organization that inverts his and his long-term mentor's respective roles. The trust and goodwill established in a long-term mentorship can go a long way in making this sort of transition experience a positive one.

Example:

You acknowledge the importance of his personal goals. Following the meeting, you consult with the nurses, who report that he appears comfortable and capable with his own patients but struggles when called after hours for a labouring person he doesn't know. You propose to him that he give up obstetric privileges after his last patient delivers in the next 3 months. In the meantime, you tell him he is relieved of on-call responsibilities. He agrees with this proposal and expresses his appreciation.

PERSONAL CHALLENGES

Example:

You are in charge of scheduling the family medicine on-call roster for perinatal care. One evening, the labour room nurses are unable to locate a colleague, the on-call provider, who is needed urgently for an obstetric emergency. She was your assigned mentor when you first joined the hospital. You are now required to assert your role in maintaining the integrity of the on-call system. You realize that you are walking a tightrope between acting as a colleague with your former mentor and your responsibility for the on-call roster. The mentorship technique you employ is gentle inquiry: "Were you available when the nurses were calling?" "What was your plan for the nurses to get a provider at the time when you could not be found?" Your goal is to mentor a senior colleague and effect change to ensure there would never be the possibility of a lapse in coverage from the family medicine perinatal care group. You also want to preserve the important and long-standing relationship with your senior colleague. Because lapses in care invariably engender feelings of shame in physicians, the mentorship grows fraught with emotion. You are determined to act with the precision and compassion that the circumstance demands.

This situation entails a reversal in previous roles in the context of a charged situation. The attributes and skills of a good mentor inform the approach. Being supportive and "gentle," as described in this scenario, creates an environment in which a mentee (and senior colleague in this case) can acknowledge concerns and admit shortcomings. Problems that manifest as lapses in professional responsibility include depression, burnout, substance abuse, clinical overload, personal or financial problems, and more. An appropriate response is possible only if underlying issues are identified. Honesty, trust, and having the best interests of the mentee at heart all contribute to a positive resolution (Straus & Sackett, 2014).

CROSS-DISCIPLINE MENTORSHIPS

Example:

You have been providing office- and hospital-based clinical preceptorships to midwifery students from the program at a local university for many years. As she completes a rotation with you, a student asks if you would continue to mentor her. You recognize that midwives train in their own unique educational program and benefit from exposure to physicians. You also appreciate that midwifery students' knowledge improves your own practice. Knowing that this student would be a potential future colleague, you are keen, if somewhat anxious, to become a cross-discipline mentor. Based on your experience mentoring physicians, you decide to share these thoughts and feelings with the midwifery student as a step to establishing a healthy mentorship.

Multi-professional training in emergency obstetric and neonatal care has been shown to save lives and improve outcomes (Bergh et al., 2015). Mentorship is integral to improving teamwork through interprofessional collaboration. Opportunities arise for both informal and formal cross-discipline mentoring in the context of training as interprofessional teams (Ngabonzima et al.,

2020). Sharing perspectives and knowledge specific to each discipline not only enhances teamwork but also builds collective understanding and coordination. As generalists, family physicians are familiar with incorporating skills and knowledge from a broad range of sources (Handford & Hennen, 2014). This approach to learning and respect for different disciplines predisposes family doctors to engage in cross-discipline mentorships.

COMBINED CARE

Example:

You work closely with a family physician colleague who refers her pregnant patients to you for delivery. The two of you met during her residency, and the teacher-student relationship has evolved over many years into mentorship and friendship. She often calls you with questions about how to manage situations to do with the care of a particular pregnant patient before referring them. You see the role as mentor to be supportive of your colleague's wish to provide prenatal care, and you strive not only to answer her questions but to also nurture her confidence and skills. You appreciate that she is an important source of ongoing referrals for intra-partum care as the patients in your own practice grow out of their child-bearing years.

Shared perinatal care provides a great opportunity for mentorship between family physicians who provide intrapartum care and those who provide pre-natal, postpartum, and newborn care. When care is shared between midwives and consultants—whether specialist obstetricians or family physicians with a focused practice—there can be challenges to communication and relationships (Bai et al., 2008; Hatten-Masterson & Griffiths, 2009; Munro et al., 2013). The scenario for this section describes a functioning model of care that evolved from a teaching relationship based on principles of good mentorship. This kind of relationship is endorsed in an interprofessional position paper on rural obstetrics (Miller et al., 2017). Mentorship is essential to achieving some of the key outcomes provided by the multidisciplinary group that produced this paper, including . . .

- Providing high-quality perinatal care that is collaborative, patient- and family-centred, culturally sensitive, respectful, and as close to the patient's home as possible
- Providing access to an integrated perinatal care system to all patients
- Implementing innovative interprofessional models
- Including collaborative practice in the training of midwives, nurses, and physicians, as well as the necessary clinical skills and competencies
- Valuing generalist skills in perinatal care, surgery, and anesthesia training programs
- Supporting ongoing, collaborative, interprofessional continuing education and patient safety programs

Conclusion

The "Quadruple Aim" in healthcare consists of . . .

- Enhancing patient experience
- Improving the health of the population
- Reducing costs
- Improving the work life of healthcare providers (Bodenheimer & Sinsky, 2014)

Capable mentorship plays a powerful part in improving the work experience of providers, which is essential to improving the patient experience (Ngabonzim et al., 2020). It thus contributes to two of these aims.

Readers who are family physicians will recognize that many of the skills and techniques of mentoring build on core competencies of the discipline. Focusing on the needs of the mentee is akin to being patient-centred. Awareness of context and community is important both for patient care and mentorship. A broad, generalist orientation and collaborative approach may help sustain relationships between patients, colleagues, and mentees. Perinatal care demands the maintenance of a high level of skill, with constant reflection on one's practice and purposive upgrading. Mentors challenge both themselves and their mentees to strive for this excellence.

REFERENCES

Avery, D.M., Skinner, C.A., & Reed, M.D. (2019). Supporting family physician maternity care providers. Family Medicine, 51(4), 362. https://doi.org/10.22454/FamMed.2019.636289

Bai, J., Gyaneshwar, R., & Bauman, A. (2008). Models of antenatal care and obstetric outcomes in Sydney South West: Antenatal care models. Australian & New Zealand Journal of Obstetrics & Gynaecology, 48(5), 454–461. https://doi.org/10.1111/j.1479-828X.2008.00888.x

Barreto, T.W., Eden, A., Hansen, E.R., & Peterson, L.E. (2019). Opportunities and Barriers for Family Physician Contribution to the Maternity Care Workforce. Family Medicine, 51(5), 383-388. https://doi.org/10.22454/FamMed.2019.845581.

Baugh, S., & Fagenson-Eland, E. (2008). Formal mentoring programs: a "poor cousin to informal relationships? In B.R. Ragins, & K.E. Kram The handbook of mentoring at work: Theory, research, and practice (pp. 249-272). SAGE Publications, Inc.

Belle Brown, J., Thorpe, C., Paquette-Warren, J., Stewart, M., & Kasperski, J. (2012). The mentoring needs of trainees in family practice. Education for Primary Care, 23(3), 196–203. https://doi.org/10.1080/14739879.2012.11494103

Bergh, A.M., Baloyi, S., & Pattinson, R.C. (2015). What is the impact of multi-professional emergency obstetric and neonatal care training? Best practice & research. Clinical Obstetrics & Gynecology, 29(8), 1028–1043. https://doi.org/10.1016/j.bpobgyn.2015.03.017https://podcasts.google.com/feed/aHR0cHM6Ly9mZWVVkcy5zaW-1wbGVjYXN0LmNvbS81NG5BR2NJbA/episode/NmE3ZjUxMzgtNjhkMS00MTliLWFlMGEtY2Y2NDgzNTdhZWY0?hl=en-CA&ved=2ahUKEwj02bvImaX1AhWoj4kEHeNQBbgQieUEegQIFhAF&ep=6

Berk, R.A., Berg, J., Mortimer, R., Walton-Moss, B., & Yeo, T.P. (2005). Measuring the effectiveness of faculty mentoring relationships. Academic Medicine, Journal of the Association of American Medical Colleges. https://podcasts.google.com/feed/aHR0cHM6Ly9mZWVVkcy5zaW1wbGVjYXN0LmNvbS81NG5BR2NJbA/episode/NmE3ZjUxMzgtNjhkMS00MTliLWFlMGEtY2Y2NDgzNTdhZWY0?hl=en-CA&ved=2ahUKEwj02bvImaX1AhWoj4kEHeNQBbgQieUEegQIFhAF&ep=6, 80(1), 66–71. https://doi.org/10.1097/00001888-200501000-00017

Biringer, A., Abells, D., Boro, J., Permaul, J.A., Sinha, S., & Graves, L. (2019). Enhanced skills training in family medicine maternity care. Canadian Family Physician, 65(12), e531-e537. http://www.cfp.ca/content/65/12/e531.abstract

Biringer, A., Forte, M., Tobin, A., Shaw, E., & Tannenbaum, D. (2018). What influences success in family medicine maternity care education programs? Canadian Family Physician, 64(5), e242-e248. Retrieved from http://www.cfp.ca/content/64/5/e242.abstract

Bodenheimer, T., & Sinsky, C. (2014). From triple to quadruple aim: care of the patient requires care of the provider. Annals of Family Medicine, 12(6), 573–576. https://doi.org/10.1370/afm.1713

Carroll, J., Brown, J., & Reid, A. (1995). Female family physicians in obstetrics: Achieving personal balance. Canadian Medical Association Journal, 153(9), 1283–1289.

Coombs, A.A.T., & King, R.K. (2005). Workplace discrimination: experiences of practicing physicians. Journal of the National Medical Association, 97(4), 467-477. https://pubmed.ncbi.nlm.nih.gov/15868767

Ericsson, K.A. (2008). Deliberate practice and acquisition of expert performance: a general overview. Academic Emergency Medicine, 15(11), 988–994. https://doi.org/10.1111/j.1553-2712.2008.00227.x

Fnais, N., Soobiah, C., Chen, M.H., Lillie, E., Perrier, L., Tashkhandi, M., Straus, S.E., Mamdani, M., Al-Omran, M., & Tricco, A.C. (2014). Harassment and Discrimination in Medical Training: A Systematic Review and Meta-Analysis. Academic Medicine, 89(5), 817-827. doi: 10.1097/ACM.0000000000000200

Frei, E., Stamm, M., & Buddeberg-Fischer, B. (2010). Mentoring programs for medical students—a review of the PubMed literature 2000-2008. BioMed Central Medical Education, 10, 32. https://doi.org/10.1186/1472-6920-10-32

Godwin, M., Hodgetts, G., Seguin, R., & MacDonald, S. (2002). The Ontario Family Medicine Residents Cohort Study: factors affecting residents' decisions to practice obstetrics. Canadian Medical Association Journal, 166(2), 179-184. http://www.cmaj.ca/content/166/2/179.abstract

Goldstein, J.T., Hartman, S.G., Meunier, M.R., Panchal, B., Pecci, C. C., Zink, N.M., & Shields, S.G. (2018). Supporting Family Physician Maternity Care Providers. Family Medicine, 50(9), 662-671. https://doi.org/10.22454/FamMed.2018.325322.

Handford, C., & Hennen, B. (2014). The gentle radical. Canadian Family Physician, 60(1):20-23.

Hatten-Masterson, S.J., & Griffiths, M.L. (2009). SHARED maternity care: enhancing clinical communication in a private maternity hospital setting. The Medical journal of Australia, 190(S11), S150–S151. https://doi.org/10.5694/j.1326-5377.2009.tb02624.x

Holbeche, L. (1996). Peer mentoring: the challenges and opportunities. Career Development International, 1(7), 24–27.

Homer. (1903). In Mackail J.W. (Ed.), The Odyssey. London: J. Murray.

Jackson, V.A., Palepu, A., Szalacha, L., Caswell, C., Carr, P.L., & Inui, T. (2003). "Having the right chemistry": a qualitative study of mentoring in academic medicine. Academic Medicine, 78(3), 328–334. https://doi.org/10.1097/00001888-200303000-00020

Jacobi, M. (1991). Mentoring and undergraduate academic success: A literature review. Review of Educational Research, 61(4), 505–532. https://doi.org/10.3102/00346543061004505

Jordan, K., Fenwick, J., Slavin, V., Sidebotham, M., & Gamble, J. (2013). Level of burnout in a small population of Australian midwives. Women and Birth: Journal of the Australian College of Midwives, 26(2), 125–132. https://doi.org/10.1016/j.wombi.2013.01.002

Kammeyer-Mueller, J., & Judge, T.A. (2008). A quantitative review of mentoring research: Test of a model. Journal of Vocational Behaviour, 72(3), 269-283. https://http://dx.doi.org/10.1016/j.jvb.2007.09.006

Koppula, S., Brown, J.B., & Jordan, J.M. (2011). Experiences of family physicians who practice primary care obstetrics in groups. Journal of Obstetrics and Gynaecology Canada, 33(2), 121-126. https://https://doi.org/10.1016/S1701-2163(16)34796-X

Koppula, S., Brown, J.B., & Jordan, J.M. (2012). Experiences of family medicine residents in primary care obstetrics training. Family Medicine, 44(3), 178–182. PMID: 22399480

Koppula, S., Brown, J.B., & Jordan, J.M. (2014). Teaching primary care obstetrics. Canadian Family Physician, 60(3), e180-e186. http://www.cfp.ca/content/60/3/e180.abstract

Marcdante, K., & Simpson, D. (2018). Choosing when to advise, coach, or mentor. Journal of Graduate Medical Education, 10(2), 227–228. https://doi.org/10.4300/JGME-D-18-00111.1

McManus, S., & Russell, J. (2008). Peer mentoring relationships. In B.R. Ragins, & K.E. Kram, The handbook of mentoring at work: Theory, research, and practice. SAGE Publications, p273-298.

Miller, K.J., Couchie, C., Ehman, W., Graves, L., Grzybowski, S., & Medves, J. (2017). No. 282-Rural Maternity Care. Journal of Obstetrics and Gynaecology Canada, 39(12), e558-e565. https://10.1016/j.jogc.2017.10.019

Munro, S., Kornelsen, J., & Grzybowski, S. (2013). Models of maternity care in rural environments: barriers and attributes of interprofessional collabouration with midwives. Midwifery, 29(6), 646–652. https://doi.org/10.1016/j.midw.2012.06.004

Ngabonzima, A., Kenyon, C., Hategeka, C., Utuza, A.J., Banguti, P.R., Luginaah, I., & F Cechetto, D. (2020). Developing and implementing a novel mentorship model (4+1) for maternal, newborn and child health in Rwanda. BioMed Central Health Services Research, 20(1), 924. https://doi.org/10.1186/s12913-020-05789-z

Pololi, L.H., Evans, A.T., Gibbs, B.K., Krupat, E., Brennan, R.T., & Civian, J.T. (2013). The experience of minority faculty who are underrepresented in medicine, at 26 representative U.S. medical schools. Academic Medicine, 88(9), 1309-1314. doi: 10.1097/ACM.0b013e31829eefff

P-Sontag, L., Vappie, K., & Wanberg, C. (2008). The practice of mentoring: Menttium Corporation. In B.R. Ragins, & K.E. Kram. The handbook of mentoring at work: Theory, research, and practice. SAGE Publications, (p593-616).

Quaas, A.M., Berkowitz, L.R., & Tracy, E.E. (2009). Evaluation of a formal mentoring program in an obstetrics and gynecology residency training program: resident feedback and suggestions. Journal of Graduate Medical Education, 1(1), 132–138. https://doi.org/10.4300/01.01.0022

Sambunjak, D., Straus, S.E., & Marušić, A. (2006). Mentoring in academic medicine: a systematic review. The Journal of the American Medical Association, 296(9), 1103–1115. https://doi.org/10.1001/jama.296.9.1103

Sambunjak, D., Straus, S.E., & Marušić, A. (2010). A systematic review of qualitative research on the meaning and characteristics of mentoring in academic medicine. Journal of General Internal Medicine, 25(1), 72–78. https://doi.org/10.1007/s11606-009-1165-8

Simpson, J., & Weiner, E. (1989). The Oxford English Dictionary. Clarendon Press.

Standing Committee on Postgraduate Medical and Dental Education. (1998). Supporting doctors and dentists at work: an enquiry into mentoring. London: SCOPME.

Straus, S.E., & Sackett, D.L. (2014). Mentorship in Academic Medicine. John Wiley & Sons. p. 1-34.

Stubbs, B., Krueger, P., White, D., Meaney, C., Kwong, J., & Antao, V. (2016). Mentorship perceptions and experiences among academic family medicine faculty: Findings from a quantitative, comprehensive work-life and leadership survey. Canadian Family Physician, 62(9), e531–e539.

Tracy, E.E., Jagsi, R., Starr, R., & Tarbell, N.J. (2004). Outcomes of a pilot faculty mentoring program. American Journal of Obstetrics and Gynecology, 191(6), 1846–1850. https://doi.org/10.1016/j.ajog.2004.08.002

Williams, L.L., Levine J.B., Malhotra, S., & Holtzheimer, P. (2004). The Good-Enough Mentoring Relationship. Academic Psychiatry, 28(2):111-5. doi: 10.1176/appi.ap.28.2.111

Chapter 8

TEACHING PERINATAL CARE TO
THE UNINTERESTED LEARNER

Perle Feldman, Hannah Shenker

Siobhan is a 1st-year family medicine resident in a family medicine peri-natal care rotation. She has just finished a rotation in labour and delivery with the obstetrics and gynecology team. Siobhan is a strong resident who generally does very well on her evaluations. When applying to residency, she hesitates between the Royal College emergency medicine program and family medicine program with an enhanced skills year in emergency medicine. In the end, she chooses family medicine because her partner wants to work in a remote community, and it seems more practical. She has been quite vocal about how perinatal care is "not for her." She has lobbied vociferously for being allowed to switch out her perinatal care rotation for "something more useful." She complains about the hours, the overnight call, and the rotation's general uselessness given that she will never practise perinatal care in her life.

When you come in for your call and ask where she is, the charge nurse says dryly: "Not here. She's never here unless we page her." You page the resident and find her in the lounge, where she is reading her ACLS manual. Feeling a "when I was a resident" moment coming on, you stop to consider how you can best teach this learner.

Most family physicians who choose to provide perinatal care do so for the love of the discipline and the privilege of following patients through pregnancy, delivery, and the postnatal phase. These perinatal care providers are often passionate teachers who look to pass their art on to the next generation of family physicians. How can these dedicated teachers approach the learner who is reluctant, uninterested, or fearful of perinatal care?

The reasons behind residents' reluctance to participate in perinatal care are many, though often based in anxiety or fear of the unknown. The unpredictable nature of childbirth can be anxiety-provoking. Negative experiences in labour and delivery as medical students—whether due to a toxic work environment or having witnessed a dramatic event—also contribute to resident reluctance to participate in perinatal care (Bédard et al., 2006). In addition, the common misconception that perinatal care is incompatible with a reasonable work-life balance leads to residents' avoidance and disinterest in the field.

This chapter will address how to work with the uninterested learner. Although this applies mainly to the family medicine training environment where learners may choose not to practise perinatal care after graduation, the principles and techniques can be applied to learning in all disciplines. We will . . .

- Introduce educational techniques to foster motivation
- Describe some general approaches to effectively teach uninterested learners in perinatal care

Fostering Motivation in the Uninterested Learner

USING MOTIVATION THEORY TO MOTIVATE

Motivation is a crucial concept in the approach to an uninterested learner in any field of education, including in teaching perinatal care. In education, high motivation is a predictor for academic success, continuation in the field of study, and general well-being. Motivation can be further characterized as either intrinsic or extrinsic:

- Intrinsic motivation describes when a person pursues an activity for personal interest or enjoyment
- Extrinsic motivation describes when a person pursues an activity for a separable outcome, i.e., to obtain a reward or to avoid a loss (Kusurkar et al., 2011)

Learners who are intrinsically motivated are autonomous and self-determined. They often have a predetermined interest in the subject at hand and are eager to learn. The uncommitted learner can be motivated extrinsically by the pressures or expectations of other—but they can also come to recognize the importance of the study and even learn to value it. In this way, an uninterested learner who is initially motivated only by external pressures—like the need to pass an exam—can become intrinsically motivated as the lesson's value becomes more apparent. This is an important concept to keep in mind when approaching the uninterested learner. A skilled teacher will not put aside the "anti-partum" learner but will assist them to internalize their motivation by ensuring adequate clinical exposure, strong role-modelling, and a supportive learning environment.

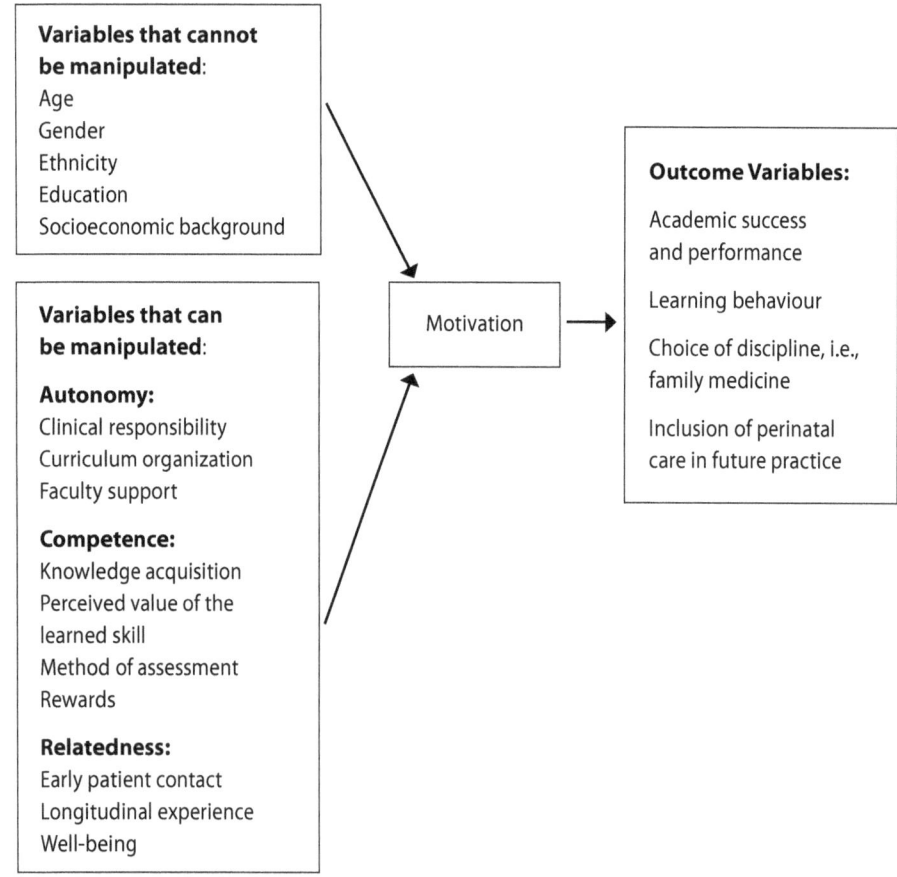

FIGURE 1: ADAPTED FOR FAMILY MEDICINE FROM "DIAGRAMMATIC REPRESENTATION OF EMPIRICALLY FOUND VARIABLES THAT AFFECT MOTIVATION OR THAT ARE AFFECTED BY MOTIVATION." (KUSURKAR ET AL., 2011)

Figure 1 demonstrates factors that can affect motivation in health professions education and its outcomes variables, such as academic success, learning behaviours, and career choices. The authors classify the factors affecting motivation as those that can be manipulated and those that cannot. Factors such as age, gender, and personal background are examples of variables that cannot be manipulated. Variables related to autonomy, competence, and "relatedness," on the other hand, can be affected by curriculum choices and teaching approaches. The authors of the diagram from which this one is adapted suggest that motivation can be a dependent variable in medical education: it can be influenced by curriculum changes or teachers' actions, too. For example, learners who are given more autonomy in clinical tasks or who have the opportunity to forge more meaningful relationships with patients over time may become more intrinsically motivated. In this way, a challenging, uninterested learner can become more motivated and learn through their enjoyment and their own improved academic performance.

Example:

Think back to Siobhan, the family medicine resident introduced at the beginning of this chapter who has little interest in perinatal care and has openly voiced her discontent. Siobhan is a highly capable resident who is extrinsically motivated by the desire to succeed academically. Take the opportunity to offer Siobhan increased autonomy in the care of perinatal patients, as she is capable—despite being uncommitted. Do not label her as challenging, but as teachable. Through increased autonomy, she will become increasingly competent and motivated.

Go on to increase the "relatedness" of the rotation by pointing out the pertinence of various skills learned in perinatal care to other fields of medicine. Siobhan is interested in emergency medicine, so use the management of obstetrical emergencies to reframe scenarios she may encounter in the emergency department or family medicine clinic. As she becomes more autonomous, competent, and understanding of the transferability of the skills she is learning in perinatal care, you may even instill some of your love of perinatal care in this otherwise uninterested learner.

USING CURRICULUM TO MOTIVATE

Starting at the Beginning: Motivating Undergraduate Medical Students in Perinatal Care

Interest in practising perinatal care develops early in a learner's training. To foster motivation, the following factors should be considered:

- Role-modelling plays a crucial role in shaping medical students' interest in perinatal care and their decisions as to whether to pursue it
- Family medicine teachers should be involved in undergraduate education in perinatal care
- Family physicians play an important role in perinatal care. Medical students should therefore be given the opportunity to work with family medicine preceptors as role models.
- There is value in providing an academic environment in which clinical teaching time is protected and prioritized for attending staff in family medicine and perinatal care (Bédard et al., 2006; Biringer et al., 2012)

In a program implementing the above strategies, 1st-year medical students participated in a continuity care experience with family physician preceptors and pregnant patients. Through this longitudinal, family-centred health experience, the students gained knowledge about the management of pregnancy and the family physician's role in perinatal care. These students demonstrated better obstetrical knowledge and interest in perinatal care at the end of the program (Westra et al., 2008).

The Next Step: Addressing Perinatal Care in Postgraduate Education

Two important factors that affect the ability of postgraduate programs to foster motivation in their family medicine learners with respect to perinatal care are . . .

- Challenges to recruiting and maintaining faculty
- Many learners in the program have no intention of practising perinatal care

A survey of Canadian family medicine residency programs attempted to determine the scope of residents' training in family medicine perinatal care. In general, program directors cited dynamic, enthusiastic, and dedicated faculty as their programs' most significant strengths. They identified their biggest challenge to be the maintenance of family physician interest in intrapartum care and the recruitment of faculty to provide it. Another major challenge was residents' lack of interest in perinatal care and the resulting difficulty in getting them to attend the births of patients from their practice (Biringer et al., 2009).

Factors related to success in teaching perinatal care include . . .

- Adequate clinical exposure for learners
- Financial and leadership support of the perinatal education program
- Strong role-modelling
- Supportive hospital environments
- Dedicated family medicine perinatal care providers (Biringer et al., 2018)

Furthermore, to motivate family medicine residents to practise perinatal care, it is important to address the culture of perinatal care in teaching hospitals. Residents will be inspired and motivated by learning environments where family physicians are respected as pivotal members of the healthcare team. These learners are further encouraged when they observe their preceptors engaged professionally in a collaborative environment, with other health disciplines that value the knowledge, skills, and contributions of family physician perinatal care providers (Biringer et al., 2018).

USING ROLE-MODELLING TO MOTIVATE

When family medicine residents are given the opportunity to work directly with physician role models who practice full-scope perinatal care, it helps them imagine themselves providing this aspect of comprehensive care (Biringer et al., 2018). Role-modelling is an essential component of medical education because it facilitates learning and helps trainees develop their professional identities. Effective physician role models demonstrate the following:

- Personal qualities:
    - Strong interpersonal skills
    - A positive outlook
    - Commitment to excellence and growth
    - Integrity
    - Leadership skills

- Teaching approaches:
    - The establishment of rapport with learners
    - Developing specific teaching philosophies and methods
    - Committing to the growth of learners (Wright & Carrese, 2002)

The quality of teaching can be improved by addressing how trainees learn from role models. Learners internalize and make sense of what they see when learning from role models. This enables them to reproduce observed behaviours. (Horsburgh & Ippolito, 2018).

Another framework that describes role-modelling is illustrated in Fig. 2.

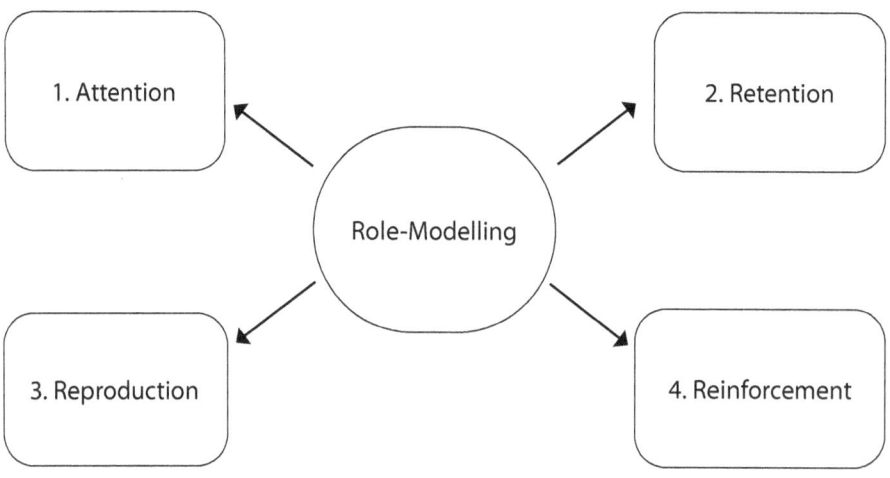

FIGURE 2: FOUR CONDITIONS NECESSARY FOR EFFECTIVE ROLE-MODELLING.
(BANDURA, 1977)

Four Conditions Necessary for Effective Role-Modelling

Attention. The trainee attends to what should be learned by observing the role model. Their learning is enhanced when they are not only physically present but when they are actively *in* the clinical encounter. Attention is also enhanced when learners observe behaviour that aligns with their view of what is important about being a doctor. Continuity of exposure to role models maintains learners' attention.

Example:

You have been assigned the same 1st-year resident for the fourth time while on call for family medicine obstetrics. The resident still appears uncomfortable being on call and tells you that they are quite nervous about the shift ahead. You make a point at the start of the shift to encourage the learner to observe what you do and ensure they feel included during the clinical encounters.

While managing the patient's second stage of labour, you say to the learner: "Pay attention to how I coach the patient and her partner. Also, I could use your involvement by having you hold the leg and put the warm compresses on the perineum."

Retention. Learners need to internalize and retain what they observe during clinical encounters. Retention involves processes in which they mentally rehearse the behaviour or actions that are to be reproduced. Learners will retain more when the preceptor provides insight into their thought processes, thereby enabling trainees to understand the reasoning behind their behaviours. When teachers share their own clinical reflections with trainees, the experience becomes more meaningful and retention is improved.

Talk through your clinical decision-making processes with learners. After a clinical encounter, think out loud. Review your differential diagnoses and concerns. Check off pertinent positive and negative findings out loud so that learners understand why you have ruled certain diagnoses in or out. Talk them through your management plan and how you will go about putting it into practice. When learners are involved in their preceptors' processes of reflection, their engagement and retention is improved.

Example:

After a delivery with the 1st-year family medicine resident introduced above, you perform the newborn exam together. After finding a subtle hip click, you review the importance of removing a newborn's diaper before assessing for hip stability.

Reproduction. Learners benefit from the opportunity to reproduce behaviours by converting the information obtained from attention and retention processes into action. Providing learners with opportunities for hands-on practice will significantly impact their retention—as well as their enjoyment—of clinical encounters.

Example:

You are supervising the inexperienced resident mentioned earlier, waiting for a fully dilated primiparous patient to start pushing. You decide to use this time to review the manoeuvres you have used in other deliveries during the shift. When the time comes for the patient to deliver, you facilitate the learner's delivery of the baby.

Reinforcement. Role-modelling can reinforce behaviours—either positively or negatively. When observing clinical encounters, trainees not only learn directly from the behaviour they witness, but also indirectly from others' reactions to this behaviour. In this way, learners may choose to avoid certain behaviours based on the negative reactions or outcomes to it they observe.

Example:

While rounding on the postpartum unit on the last day of the resident's perinatal care rotation, you do a newborn exam and counsel the parents while the learner observes. After the encounter, you ask the learner how they think it went and whether they could provide some feedback on the interaction in terms of what worked and what did not. The learner responds by saying that they noticed the parents were listening attentively and the nurse was nodding her head in agreement with your proposed discharge plan. By observing the positive impact of this interaction on the patients and your colleague, the effectiveness of your approach was reinforced for the resident.

General Approaches to the Uninterested Learner

In the following section, various approaches to engaging the learner who is uninterested in perinatal care are reviewed.

SHARING THE PASSION OF INTRAPARTUM CARE

Family medicine residents benefit from a work environment where preceptors model a passion for their art (Biringer et al., 2018). Perinatal care providers can help learners appreciate the privileged role of the family physician, who follows a pregnancy from conception through childbirth and then supports families through the challenges of the postnatal period and raising a child. They have the opportunity to show learners a practice that involves challenging technical skills and the forging of longstanding relationships with patients and their families.

While not all family medicine residents might be expected to include intrapartum care in their future careers, they should all learn that perinatal care is an integral part of family medicine. Family physicians are uniquely prepared to provide continuity of perinatal care within a comprehensive biopsychosocial model of primary care (Biringer et al., 2012). This approach to patient care is professionally gratifying and attractive to learners when role-modelled effectively.

Example:

You are on call in the delivery room and are reviewing the active patient board with the resident, who is starting her shift. Upon discussing a primiparous patient who has been progressing nicely all day, the resident's face lights up. "Oh, I know that woman—I met her last night when she presented to triage in latent phase. We sent her home with instructions. It looks like she came back in active labour!" You ask the resident to go check on the patient to see how she is managing her contractions and progressing. Judging the resident capable, you ask them to manage the patient overnight—but to call you with any questions or concerns they have. A few hours later, the resident calls you to tell you that the patient is fully dilated with a strong urge to push. You arrive to find the patient pushing well and the delivery imminent. The resident has clearly formed a close bond with the couple, and they are able to joke and discuss baby names between contractions. The delivery goes smoothly, and the newborn is placed skin-to-skin. You observe the resident taking in the joy of the new parents. As you are filling in the paperwork, the resident tells you that this was the highlight of her rotation so far. You agree that it was a beautiful birth and say simply, "I am so lucky I get to do this every day and so glad you were here to enjoy this moment."

MYTH BUSTERS: TRUTH, LIES, AND FAMILY MEDICINE PERINATAL CARE

Learners may hold preconceived notions, or myths, about practising perinatal care following training and therefore chose not to do so. Here we break down some common misconceptions about practising perinatal care.

Myth #1: Obstetrical Practice Will Take Over Your Life

It is important to show residents models of reasonable work-life balance in perinatal care and address their concerns about the impact of practice on their personal lives. Role-modelling is critical here—probably the most effective educational tool in our arsenal.

Many family medicine residents come into residency with an interest in intrapartum care, but are concerned about its impact on their own quality of life. It is vital to make the truths about perinatal care in family medicine explicit to these learners. This may have already been undermined by their other experiences in undergraduate medical education. We know that learners with access to family medicine perinatal care providers as role models during clerkship are more likely to see perinatal care as a doable, less frightening, and more viable part of their medical practice compared to those without that exposure (Graves et al., 2012; Bédard et al., 2006.). Family physicians who continue to practise intrapartum care do so because their particular on-call system allows them to have a reasonable quality of life (Dove et al., 2017). Residents should be exposed to role models who have achieved an appropriate work-life balance while providing intrapartum care. They should be provided with various ways to integrate perinatal care into family medicine in a balanced and sustainable manner. These could include call groups and shiftwork in labour and delivery (Biringer et al., 2018).

Example:

It has been a busy night in the delivery room on call with a family medicine resident. You have just finished the delivery of one of your own patients. Following the delivery, you ask the resident about their future. "You seem to have a real talent for perinatal care. What are your plans for practice?"

"I like perinatal care," says the resident. "I like the acuity and the challenge, and I love the patient population, but I worry I won't be able to have a balanced family life with the calls and the night work."

You answer, "Many family docs who include perinatal care in their practice work the same number of hours as those who don't. If you have a good call group whom you trust and who are respectful of your personal values, it can be perfectly compatible with family life. Some family physicians who provide perinatal care will come to the hospital to deliver all their patients, while others work in call groups and will defer deliveries to the on-call physician. Practising perinatal care in family medicine offers a lot of flexibility in shared on-call responsibilities. If you're interested, we can talk about it more."

Myth #2: Malpractice Claims Frequently Occur in Perinatal Care

Another common concern among learners is the fear of malpractice claims related to intrapartum care. In reality, malpractice claims are quite low for family doctors providing perinatal care (Larimore & Sapolsky, 1995). Residents can be reassured that low-risk obstetrical practice is well within the scope of general family medicine. Malpractice insurance premiums are less costly for family physicians practising perinatal care as compared to specialists. In addition, family physicians tend to forge longstanding relationships with their patients and demonstrate strong communication skills, a practice that is well-documented as the best protection against malpractice claims (Levinson et al., 1997).

Myth #3: Obstetrical Practice Is Scary and Unpredictable

It is important to remind residents that most deliveries go well and that family physicians are specialists in physiologic birth, a natural process that can be practised with a low rate of intervention. Though residents should be trained to manage obstetrical emergencies, they need to be reminded that these are rare occurrences.

Practitioners who enjoy procedural skills and the hospital's interprofessional environment can find this in the delivery room. Therefore, teachers should share the thrill and excitement of intrapartum care with their trainees, all the while reassuring them that family physicians can develop the skillset to competently manage this very exciting work.

Example:

You are attending the birth of a multiparous woman in active labour while supervising a nervous family medicine resident. The patient is labouring without epidural anesthesia and has been encouraged to mobilize. She manages her contractions by vocalizing loudly and dancing around the room as a nurse performs intermittent auscultation. The patient has chosen to forego the hospital gown, since she finds it constricting. You are calm and waiting for the patient to express an urge to push. The resident is obviously uncomfortable with all the noise and the difficulty in consistently monitoring the fetal heart.

The patient suddenly bears down, and the head emerges with a tight nuchal cord. The resident panics. You calmly take over, performing a somersault manoeuvre, delivering the baby with cord intact. You turn to the resident and say, "You, too, can learn to readily do this manoeuvre when you come upon this circumstance."

APPLYING THE SKILLS AND KNOWLEDGE ACQUIRED IN INTRAPARTUM CARE TO BROAD-SCOPE FAMILY MEDICINE

Another approach to the uninterested learner is to demonstrate the value inherent in the skills they will learn in perinatal care, how they will inevitably manage perinatal patients in various settings outside of the delivery room, and how the skills learned in perinatal care can carry over to a variety of domains.

Example:

You and the resident are called down to the emergency room, where a patient has arrived, fully dilated and pushing. You help them on to the gurney, where they end up delivering on their side. Following the delivery, you debrief with this resident, who has no intention of practising intrapartum care. You recount stories from previous trainees who delivered babies in unusual circumstances. With a solid foundation from their family medicine residency, including hands-on exposure to labouring patients, they developed the necessary skill set to deliver a baby.

You describe how these emergency room, community clinic, and parking lot deliveries are different than the patient delivering in the lithotomy position under regional anesthesia.

Generally, this will catch residents' attention—eyes wide open with intrigue—and convince them of the importance of this rotation.

In addition to the capacity to attend to a precipitous delivery in a variety of settings, it is important for all family physicians to develop an approach to conditions like antepartum hemorrhage, preterm labour, and hypertensive pregnancy disorders. These conditions are examples of obstetrical complications that present outside of the labour and delivery room and which are therefore pertinent to all primary care providers. Through these types of concrete examples, we can demonstrate to reluctant learners that the skills learned in perinatal care are pertinent to a broader range of practice settings.

Below are some examples of priority topics in teaching perinatal care that can be presented as pertinent to family medicine in the non-obstetrical setting—for example, in emergency medicine, rural practice, or the urban office setting. The bottom line is that nothing is irrelevant to a family medicine learner.

Postpartum Hemorrhage

Precipitous delivery is a risk factor for postpartum hemorrhage, so it follows that patients who have unplanned deliveries in an ambulance or emergency room are at higher risk. When this occurs outside of the labour and delivery room, the care provider does not benefit from a team of nurses and physician colleagues who have repeatedly practised the management algorithm. Therefore, it is important for emergency room and rural attending physicians to be aware of the management of postpartum hemorrhage in order to be able to guide the team to stabilize patients who experience it. Additionally, the skills learned in the management of antepartum hemorrhage, postpartum hemorrhage, and disseminated intravascular coagulation can be carried over to the management of hemorrhages in general.

Preterm Labour

Preterm labour is often unexpected. Patients who live in communities without perinatal care services will travel to their planned delivery site as they approach term. Should they present in preterm labour, it will be up to the rural physician to stabilize these patients for transfer—or potentially manage the delivery and premature infant themselves.

Perineal Repair

The repair of perineal lacerations is a common procedure in perinatal care. The learner who is competent at these difficult repairs will be that much more skilled at any other laceration repair that may come their way.

Teaching Tip

Take the time to allow learners to develop a hands-on approach to perineal repair. Discuss how knowing how to suture a second-degree perineal laceration can be useful in repairing other sorts of complex wounds where you must identify different tissues, match like to like, and close the dead space without strangulating the tissues. In this way, the skills learned in perineal repair are transferable to the management of soft tissue injuries in a variety of settings.

Hypertensive Disorders in Pregnancy

Preeclampsia symptoms are not always identifiable as a hypertensive disorder of pregnancy, and may present to the emergency room or family medicine clinic as a migraine, gastrointestinal problem, cardiovascular compromise, or seizure. Family physicians must remain vigilant when seeing pregnant or postpartum patients who may present with symptoms of gestational hypertension without recognizing it as a pregnancy complication.

Treating Other Medical Problems During Pregnancy

Pregnant patients will present with other illnesses in a variety of primary care settings. They will often be concerned about the impact of their medical problem and its treatment on their unborn or breastfed infant. Therefore, family physicians should understand the special considerations involved in treating any medical conditions in the pregnant or breastfeeding patient.

Interprofessional Care

During their perinatal care experiences, residents have the opportunity to participate in interprofessional teams that can include family physicians, obstetricians, midwives, nurses, social workers, and lactation consultants, among others. The skills residents acquire in effective teamwork, communication, and professionalism will carry over to the various medical settings where they will practice in the future.

The Doctor-Patient Relationship

Perinatal care provides the opportunity to learn about the longitudinal doctor-patient relationships that are an essential part of family medicine.

Teaching Tip

When seeing a postpartum patient with a resident, explicitly discuss the patient's psychosocial background and their "story." Invite learners into your unique, longstanding doctor-patient relationship by telling them about the patient's background when you first discussed contraception options in her teen years, how you have supported her as a perinatal care provider, and how you are now caring for her during her postpartum visit, along with her baby. Family medicine residents are motivated by continuity of care and the opportunity to forge longstanding relationships with patients.

PERINATAL CARE AS A FUNDAMENTAL SKILL IN FAMILY MEDICINE

Finally, when all else fails, preceptors can approach learners pragmatically. Perinatal care is part of the family medicine curriculum and residents must attain competency in these fundamental skills to become a licensed family physician. The uninterested learner may be reluctant, but they will need to master the priority topics in perinatal care to achieve certification in family medicine.

Example:

It's a slow day in labour and delivery. There are two 2nd-year family medicine residents hanging around without much to do. You decide to give an impromptu presentation on pre-labour rupture of membranes based on a patient seen in triage earlier that morning. You are careful to link the discussion to the College of Family Physicians' priority topics, since the residents have mentioned that they are participating in a study group for their upcoming certification exams. After the presentation, you give them a few practice exam questions to answer. This will underline the importance of the perinatal care rotation for the successful passing of the certification exams—a powerful motivator for graduating residents.

Conclusion

When faced with the uninterested resident, teachers can use a variety of techniques to engage them in perinatal care. Postgraduate programs should harness their enthusiastic and dedicated teachers to role-model and engage in other motivational techniques, not only to help reluctant learners achieve basic competencies, but to engage some as future providers of perinatal care.

REFERENCES

Bandura, A. (1977). Social learning theory. Prentice Hall.

Bédard, M.J., Berthiaume, S., Beaulieu, M.D., & Leclerc, C. (2006). Factors influencing the decision to practice obstetrics among Québec medical students: A survey. Journal of Obstetrics and Gynaecology of Canada, 28(12), 1075–82.

Biringer, A., Maxted, J., & Graves, L. (2009). Family medicine maternity care: implications for the future. A discussion paper of the Maternity and Newborn Care Committee. Mississauga, ON. College of Family Physicians of Canada.

Biringer, A., Almond, R., Dupuis, K., Graves, L., Rainsberry, P., & Wilson, L. (2012). Report of the Working Group on Family Medicine Maternity Care Training. Mississauga, ON: College of Family Physicians of Canada.

Biringer, A., Forte, M., Tobin, A., Shaw, E., & Tannenbaum, D. (2018). What influences success in family medicine maternity care education programs? Qualitative exploration. Can Fam Physician, 64(5), e242-e248.

Canadian Medical Protective Association, Ottawa (CA): CMPA. (2018). College complaints on the rise, better communication can help. Available from: www.cmpa-acpm.ca/en/advice-publications/browse-articles/2018/college-complaints-on-the-rise-better-communication-can-help

Dove, M., Dogba, M.J., & Rodríguez, C. (2017). Exploring family physicians' reasons to continue or discontinue providing intrapartum care: qualitative descriptive study. Canadian Family Physician, 63(8), e387-e393.

Graves, L., & Hutten-Czapski, P. (2006). An Approach to Maternity Care Education for Canadian Family Medicine Residents: A Discussion Paper of the Maternity and Newborn Care Committee. College of Family Physicians of Canada.

Helton, M., Skinner, B., & Denniston, C. (2003). A maternal and Child Health Curriculum for Family Practice Residents: Results of an Intervention at the University of North Carolina. Family Medicine, 35(3),174-180.

Horsburgh, J., & Ippolito, K. (2018). BioMed Central Medical Education, 18, 156.

Klein, M.C. A new role model for maternity care. (1997). Canadian Family Physician, 43(16), 23-4.

Koppula, S., Brown, J.B., & Jordan, J.M. (2012). Experiences of family medicine residents in primary care obstetrics training. Family Medicine, 44(3), 178-182.

Kusurkar, R.A., ten Cate, Th.J., Van Asperen, M., & Croiset, G. (2011). Motivation as an independent and a dependent variable in medical education: A review of the literature. Medical Teacher, 33(5), e242-e262.

Larimore, W.L., & Sapolsky, B.S. (1995). Maternity care in family medicine: economics and malpractice. Journal of Family Practice, 40(2), 153-160.

Levinson, W., Roter, D.L., Mullooly, J.P., Dull, V.T., & Frankel, R.M. (1997). Physician-patient communication. The relationship with malpractice claims among primary care physicians and surgeons. Journal of the American Medical Association, 277(7), 553-9.

Ruderman, J., Holzapfel, S.G., Carroll, J.C., & Cummings, S. (1999). Obstetrics anyone? How family medicine residents' interests changed. Canadian Family Physician, 45, 638-647.

Westra, W., Haller, I.R., Adams, J., Peterson, B.J., Pearson, J. (2008). Early introduction to pregnancy care and delivery for medical students. Family Medicine, 40(1), 17-23.

Wright, S., & Carrese, J. (2002). Excellence in role-modelling: insight and perspectives from the pros. Canadian Medical Association Journal, 167, 638–43.

Chapter 9

COMPETENCY-BASED EDUCATION

David Tannenbaum, Evan Tannenbaum

Dr. Pierre Tremblay, when he is on-call covering the labour and delivery unit, begins working with learners from the local medical school. He has been in community practice for 15 years, away from the world of medical education. He recalls focusing on learning objectives during his residency and needing to pass each rotation to successfully complete it. To assist learners to achieve their goals during their time working with him, he signs up for an online course about competency-based medical education. This chapter outlines what he learns.

Competency-Based Education (CBE)

Health professions education programs across the globe are migrating to CBE, an educational approach that focuses on the outcomes of training, i.e., the knowledge and skills—or competencies—required at the completion of training to safely meet the needs of patients and society.

Passing a clinical placement does not necessarily ensure the learner has achieved competency in the many clinical tasks and activities associated with the particular area of professional practice. CBE takes a more deliberate approach to teaching and learning by carefully selecting the learning experiences that will be most effective in helping learners acquire these necessary competencies. CBE also requires assessing learners at multiple points in time and in various clinical situations to ensure these competencies have been met (Frank et al., 2010). Rather than relying on a relatively small collection of end-of-rotation evaluations to judge a trainee's abilities, CBE relies on a larger collection of bite-sized assessments of a learner's performance in an array of clinical encounters and tasks (e.g., inducing labour, repairing a perineal tear). With frequent feedback, coaching, and assessment, learners are guided toward unsupervised practice (Holmboe et al., 2010). Through its assessment tools, the program is able to demonstrate that the trainee has met the learning goals and achieved competency for independent practice.

A CBE training program should . . .

- Outline the competencies expected to be met at completion of training
- Ensure learners are given the clinical training opportunities to acquire these competencies
- Individualize each learner's education rather than relying on a universally assigned time-based approach (e.g., month blocks)
- Adequately assess the learner and document their achievements to demonstrate that the necessary competencies were attained (Iobst et al., 2010)

ADVANTAGES AND CHALLENGES

The key advantages of CBE are . . .

- Its careful construction of learning experiences—each rotation or educational experience is selected and monitored to ascertain that the intended learning takes place
- Its effectiveness in identifying the clinical skills a learner has and has not fully mastered and the way it allows for the adjustment of training experiences to improve upon the deficits identified
- Its ability to accommodate learners' different needs given the flexibility permitted in scheduling educational experiences without tight time constraints
- Its ability to ensure, through careful assessment of the learner, that they are ready for independent practice or can intervene at early stages with support (Touchie & Ten Cate, 2016)

Challenges to CBE include . . .

- The assumption of greater responsibility by clinical teachers for monitoring learner progress
- The considerable time for coaching clinical teachers must set aside, in which they guide the learner, enhancing their performance through observation, feedback, and actionable suggestions (Landreville, et al., 2019)
- The adequate clinical exposure that must be assured learners receive, so that they may acquire the specific knowledge and skills of the discipline
- The required frequency of the use of assessment tools to document the learner's progress in each given competency and the possibility for assessment burnout, given the long lists of competencies that need to be assessed (Hawkins et al., 2015)
- The challenging nature of the administration of CBE, because learners progress at different rates and cannot always be assigned to a standard schedule

IMPLICATIONS FOR THE TEACHER

In CBE, teachers should . . .

- Know the specific competencies they are meant to teach and assess
- Set aside time to observe the learner—on multiple occasions
- Base assessments on direct observation of clinical work

  - Conduct assessments and complete standardized forms as required by each program
  - Provide effective feedback

- Determine where the learner sits on the competency spectrum—from fully dependent on the teacher's supervision to fully independent

  - Attempt to predict if the learner is capable of working independently in practice for each competency
  - Unambiguously tell them where they are on the path to independence for each competency—and how to move themselves further along (Hauer et al., 2011)

Example:

A 2nd-year family medicine resident has come to your town for a 4-week rotation in the perinatal care program. On the first day, she provides a list of competencies she has not yet mastered. These are . . .

- *The newborn exam*
- *The management of shoulder dystocia*
- *The assessment of common breastfeeding problems*

You discuss with her how she might best gain clinical experience with these specific competencies, and you assist by . . .

- *Ensuring she attends newborn rounds in the hospital*
- *Arranging that she be paged when on the labour floor to participate in the management of any obstetrical emergencies*
- *Arranging appropriate time in the labour and delivery suite and the lactation clinic for her*

You then decide to . . .

- *Monitor these experiences through a clinical activity log*
- *Review the log periodically—and adjust the assignments as needed*
- *Observe her directly in her work with patients in these (and other) clinical activities*
- *Check in with her regularly as to whether she feels she is making progress in her skill development*
- *Provide specific feedback based on input from other teachers and your direct observation to guide her in improving her performance*
- *Complete assessments—including the required forms and provide feedback to the program director on a regular basis*

See Fig. 1, which provides a summary of how to distinguish competency-based education from the more traditional time-based approach.

	Overall structure	Learning objectives	Assessment strategies	Assessment philosophy	The role of trust
Traditional curriculum	Time-based scheduling of rotations	Rotation-specific objectives that are granular and difficult to know how and when to assess	Infrequent, high-stakes, mainly pass/fail	Assumed competence based on overall ratings of learner performance	Implicit or assumed
Competency-based curriculum	Still relies on scheduled rotations meant to address specific entrustable professional activities (EPAs)	Learner selects from the discipline's list of EPAs on which to focus during the rotation	Frequent, low-stakes, meant to foster growth and reach entrustment	A picture of growth and competence is painted by repeatedly measuring the way each EPA was specifically addressed	Explicit

FIGURE 1: A COMPARISON BETWEEN COMPETENCY-BASED EDUCATION AND A MORE TRADITIONAL TIME-BASED APPROACH.

Entrustable Professional Activities (EPAs)

As CBE evolved, EPAs were created to translate competencies into clinical practice. Sometimes the terms "competency" and "EPA" are used interchangeably, which can be confusing to the teacher and learner. EPAs are descriptions of the work of a healthcare provider. Each EPA can be broken down into smaller units that further define the work of the provider, so that learner is aware of the what they need to know and which abilities they must attain (Carraccio et al., 2017; Ten Cate, 2013).

For example, perinatal care is an area of practice that can be broken down into a number of EPAs. Some of these include . . .

- Providing antenatal care
- Managing common medical disorders of pregnancy
- Managing labour in a low-risk patient

- Conducting an uncomplicated vaginal delivery
- Providing postpartum care

The EPAs—or abilities—encompass what you would expect a new colleague entering your group to be able to be "entrusted" to do independently. Each individual EPA can further be defined through more detailed descriptions of the component knowledge and abilities that permit a provider to successfully carry out that task.

For example, the EPA that pertains to the management of labour in a low-risk patient can be further broken down into . . .

- The knowledge of normal labour patterns
- The ability to assess fetal well-being
- The knowledge and skill to intervene when labour is not progressing as expected
- The ability to communicate effectively with the patient and family
- The ability to work collaboratively with the nursing team and obstetricians

The advantages of using EPAs include . . .

- The ability to break down large, complex descriptions of clinical practice into small, concrete clinical activities that can be taught, observed, and assessed
- The ability to tailor feedback to the clearly articulated component knowledge and abilities needed to manage these clinical activities effectively and safely
- The ability to assess and record performance in the most relevant aspects of day-to-day practice (Ten Cate & Taylor, 2021)

The challenges of using EPAs include . . .

- The tendency to subdivide clinical practice into an unwieldy number of EPAs
  - The resultant burden of a large number of EPAs for both the teacher and learner
- The need to adapt to this different set of expectations around teaching and evaluation (Van Loon et al., 2014)

IMPLICATIONS FOR THE TEACHER

Rather than making an overall pass/fail judgment at the end of a rotation, assessment of performance on EPAs allows a clinical teacher to make smaller, more frequent, trust-based assessments. The assessment centres on the clinical teacher's trust in the learner's ability to safely perform a given task (or EPA) and is based on what the clinical teacher sees in the moment. These small assessments of performance are accompanied by feedback and coaching—either to bring the learner to the point where they can be trusted to be independent or—if they are already at that level—to further improve and fine-tune their approach.

In CBE, fully entrusting a learner means they have achieved the expected level of knowledge and ability and are ready for independent practice (Ten Cate, 2020; Tekian et al., 2020).

Our trust in our learners is based on . . .

- Our own observations of a learner's . . .

  - Clinical performance
  - Professional behaviours, such as reliability, conscientiousness, honesty, and willingness to seek help
  - Skills in communication and collaboration

- What we are told by . . .

  - Patients
  - Other teachers
  - The training program

This implies that . . .

- Trust is built over time
- Trust may be context-specific and may vary with . . .

  - The nature and acuity of the clinical presentation
  - Patient characteristics
  - The location of the activity

- The level of trust a teacher has in a learner may vary across the spectrum of activities that comprise their area of clinical practice

– Teachers should be cautious about assuming that a learner who can be trusted in one area of clinical work can be trusted in all of them (the "halo effect")

Novice teachers—and even some who are seasoned—may have difficulty fully trusting learners and handing responsibility to them. This may relate to . . .

- A desire to maintain full control over a clinical situation
- Uncertainties about their own skills in the early practice years
- Insufficient experience with learners to know what skills should be expected of them at different stages
- Concern about being held responsible for the work conducted by learners (perhaps based on a prior negative experience)
- Concern that patients will be displeased with a learner (or themselves as a teacher)

Example:

Your 1st-year family medicine resident reports that she has discharged a postpartum patient. Based on a previous experience of observing her assess a newborn, discuss the parents' concerns, and provide appropriate guidance and follow-up, you trust her to bring significant concerns to your attention in a timely way. She has reached the level of entrustment: you believe that no further action on your part is needed to ensure she provides safe and effective care.

Entrustment Scales and Assessment Tools

Let's take a look at how to incorporate EPAs and trust in teaching and assessment.

In CBE, entrustment scales replace the traditional assessment scales with which we are familiar (Rekman et al., 2016). Entrustment scales ask us to rate the degree of trust we feel comfortable placing in learners with respect to specific clinical abilities.

Traditional assessment scales that use descriptors such as "poor" or "excellent" can be vague, unhelpful, and even demoralizing to learners. No one likes to be labelled "weak" or "below expectations"—terms such as these are value-laden and subjective—and teachers may find it difficult to rate learners below a certain level for fear of provoking a negative response. Furthermore, learners may not necessarily know what to do with the assessment they receive, as it does not offer specific guidance or lead to discussions regarding ways to improve.

Focusing on trust is a new way of offering feedback to learners. When we use trust to assess learners, we focus the judgment on the performance rather than on the individual (Ten Cate et al., 2020).

ENTRUSTMENT SCALES: FIVE LEVELS

Levels used in entrustment rating scales describe the extent to which the teacher's involvement was required to assist the learner in a given clinical situation:

- **Level 1:** The teacher had to perform the clinical activity while the learner observed
- **Level 2:** The learner required constant direction
- **Level 3:** The learner required frequent direction
- **Level 4:** The learner required minor direction (the teacher needed to be nearby "just in case")
- **Level 5:** No direction was required (the teacher did not need to be present)

Entrustment scales . . .

- Emphasize the ultimate goal of independent practice
- Are less subjective and less judgmental than traditional assessment tools and scales
- Are less prone to creating the "halo effect" than traditional assessment tools
- Avoid pejorative labels
- Make it easier for a teacher to use the full range of the rating scale (since each rating is just a report of the level of supervision that took place)
- Rely on direct observation
- Empower teachers to rely on their gut feelings, translating them into assessment scores (Dudek et al., 2019)

Entrustment is about reporting on performance in the language of trust. Stepwise, progressive acquisition of trust becomes the goal. The responsibility of the teacher is not to compare the abilities of one learner to another, but to elevate each learner to the expected level for unsupervised practice.

The challenges to teaching when using entrustment scales are . . .

- As a new method of rating performance, they may be difficult for programs and teachers to adopt and will require faculty development regarding their use
- Learners may equate the five-point entrustment scale with other, traditional assessment scales, when they are not meant to be viewed as direct equivalents
- Partial implementation of these scales leads to the need to transfer entrustment language to traditional rating scales

Examples of feedback to learners using EPAs and entrustment language:

You are on call on the labour floor and a patient has just delivered. The obstetrics resident on call with you completes the repair of the perineal laceration, and you have to provide constant guidance on suture placement and repair technique to ensure safe and effective care.

Steps in providing feedback using the language of entrustment:

- *Invite the learner to the feedback discussion at an appropriate time and location:*
  - *"Let's go to the break room to talk about that delivery."*
  - *"I think we can agree you required a lot of guidance from me during the repair."*
- *State the level of involvement required by you, the teacher, in this specific case, and elicit reflection from the learner:*
  - *"Based on what we just saw, that would be at the level of requiring constant guidance, or level 2 on our scale. Would you agree with that?"*
- *Focus on the expected target level of trust:*
  - *"No one can do a perineal repair on their own on their first day. But over time, you should be able to do repairs with greater independence.*

Our goal is to have you do the repair while I watch—which would be level 4 on our scale."

- *Create an actionable plan:*

  - *"Let's practise with the simulation model. Then, I want you to give me direction while I do the next repair."*
  - *"Once we're sure you know all the steps and techniques, I'll supervise you doing another repair, and we can see how much guidance is needed. I think we should be able reach level 4 with some practice and continued coaching."*

OTHER CONSIDERATIONS

- When giving feedback on EPAs, you may wish to point out to the learner that . . .

  - The goal of coaching is to get the learner to a specified level of independence through repeated, guided practice
  - Trust may be achieved for certain tasks or clinical activities early on, while others may take some time
  - The time to reach the expected level of trust in a given EPA varies from learner to learner, but you have confidence they can reach the level of competence expected

- You may wish to confirm your entrustment decision with case-based discussions in which you ask the learner to describe what they might do in related scenarios.

  - Example: *The resident successfully managed a shoulder dystocia with two manoeuvres—McRoberts and suprapubic pressure. You ask the resident to explain in detail what they would have done if these manoeuvres were unsuccessful.*

Conclusion

CBE is considered an advance in health professions education that ensures learners achieve prespecified levels of competence in the areas of clinical practice relevant to their needs and those of the patients and communities they will serve. In CBE, the expected competencies are defined in detail at the start of training using EPAs. Teachers carefully develop educational experiences and methods of assessment to foster learners' acquisition of these competencies, recognizing that the time required to do so will vary from learner to learner. Using direct observation, feedback, and coaching, clinical teachers guide learners toward progressive independence.

CBE holds promise in ensuring consistent, high-level care for patients and communities by ensuring that trainees graduate only when fully competent. While the benefits are clear, there may be challenges for the teacher. These relate to learning new methods of assessment, ensuring learners' exposure to appropriate training experiences and skillfully using feedback and coaching to help learners achieve their goals.

REFERENCES

Carraccio, C., Englander, R., Gilhooly, J., Mink, R., Hofkosh, D., Barone, M.A., & Holmboe, E.S. (2017). Building a framework of entrustable professional activities, *supported* by competencies and milestones, to bridge the educational continuum. Academic Medicine, 92(3), 324–330. https://doi.org/10.1097/ACM.0000000000001141

Dudek, N., Gofton, W., Rekman, J., & McDougall, A. (2019). Faculty and resident perspectives on using entrustment anchors for workplace-based assessment. Journal of Graduate Medical Education, 11(3), 287–294. https://doi.org/10.4300/JGME-D-18-01003.1

Frank, J.R., Snell, L.S., Cate, O.T., Holmboe, E.S., Carraccio, C., Swing, S.R., Harris, P., Glasgow, N.J., Campbell, C., Dath, D., Harden, R.M., Iobst, W., Long, D.M., Mungroo, R., Richardson, D.L., Sherbino, J., Silver, I., Taber, S., Talbot, M., & Harris, K.A. (2010). Competency-based medical education: Theory to practice. Medical Teacher, *32*(8), 638–645. https://doi.org/10.3109/0142159X.2010.501190

Hauer, K.E., Holmboe, E.S., & Kogan, J.R. (2011). Twelve tips for implementing tools for direct observation of medical trainees' clinical skills during patient encounters. Medical Teacher, *33*(1), 27–33. https://doi.org/10.3109/0142159X.2010.507710

Hawkins, R.E., Welcher, C.M., Holmboe, E.S., Kirk, L.M., Norcini, J.J., Simons, K.B., & Skochelak, S. E. (2015). Implementation of competency-based medical education: Are we addressing the concerns and challenges? Medical Education, 49(11), 1086–1102. https://doi.org/10.1111/medu.12831

Holmboe, E.S., Sherbino, J., Long, D.M., Swing, S.R., Frank, J.R., & for the International CBME Collabourators. (2010). The role of assessment in competency-based medical education. Medical Teacher, 32(8), 676–682. https://doi.org/10.3109/0142159X.2010.500704

Iobst, W.F., Sherbino, J., Cate, O.T., Richardson, D.L., Dath, D., Swing, S.R., Harris, P., Mungroo, R., Holmboe, E.S., & Frank, J.R., for the International CMBE Collabourators. (2010). Competency-based medical education in postgraduate medical education. Medical Teacher, 32(8), 651–656. https://doi.org/10.3109/0142159X.2010.500709

Landreville, J., Cheung, W., Frank, J., & Richardson, D. (2019). A definition for coaching in medical education. Canadian Medical Education Journal, 10(4), e109–e110. https://doi.org/10.36834/cmej.68713

Rekman, J., Gofton, W., Dudek, N., Gofton, T., & Hamstra, S.J. (2016). Entrustability Scales: Outlining Their Usefulness for Competency-based Clinical Assessment. Academic Medicine, 91(2), 186–190. https://doi.org/10.1097/ACM.0000000000001045

Tekian, A., ten Cate, O., Holmboe, E., Roberts, T., & Norcini, J. (2020). Entrustment decisions: Implications for curriculum development and assessment. Medical Teacher, 42(6), 698–704. https://doi.org/10.1080/0142159X.2020.1733506

ten Cate, O. (2013). Nuts and Bolts of Entrustable Professional Activities. Journal of Graduate Medical Education, 5(1), 157–158. https://doi.org/10.4300/JGME-D-12-00380.1

ten Cate, O. (2020). When I say … entrustability. Medical Education, *54*(2), 103–104. https://doi.org/10.1111/medu.14005

ten Cate, O., Schwartz, A., & Chen, H.C. (2020). Assessing Trainees and Making Entrustment Decisions: On the Nature and Use of Entrustment-Supervision Scales. Academic Medicine, 95(11), 1662–1669. https://doi.org/10.1097/ACM.0000000000003427

Ten Cate, O., & Taylor, D.R. (2021). The recommended description of an entrustable professional activity: AMEE Guide No. 140. Medical Teacher, 43(10), 1106–1114. https://doi.org/10.1080/0142159X.2020.1838465

Touchie, C., & ten Cate, O., (2016). The promise, perils, problems and progress of competency-based medical education. Medical Education, 50(1), 93–100. https://doi.org/10.1111/medu.12839

van Loon, K.A., Driessen, E.W., Teunissen, P.W., & Scheele, F. (2014). Experiences with EPAs, potential benefits and pitfalls. Medical Teacher, 36(8), 698–702. https://doi.org/10.3109/0142159X.2014.909588

Chapter 10

EVALUATION

Gary Viner

Dr. Joana Van Dyke and her colleagues have been working with learners in the labour and delivery unit at the local hospital for several years. Upon conclusion of each rotation at the hospital, the teachers complete evaluation forms specific to the learner's institution. In order to create a more robust system at her hospital, Dr. Van Dyke wants to learn more about basic concepts of the evaluation of learners. Also, she wants the learners to evaluate the teachers and the perinatal care rotation overall. Though she gets informal comments from learners as they finish their rotations, she feels that a detailed, anonymous system would be more revealing and accurate. To learn more about how an evaluation system could work at their hospital, she attends a course on evaluation at a national conference. This is what she learns at the sessions she attends.

The Evaluation of Learners

INTRODUCTION

In perinatal care, learners are expected to attain the skills necessary to meet the standards for the safe provision of care either as a primary provider or as one with more peripheral involvement—such as offering intercurrent or emergent care. As teachers in any domain, our goal is to assist the learner and ensure the necessary skills are acquired and maintained. It is therefore intrinsic to teaching to evaluate learners' assimilation of this information. Learner evaluation is the process of comparing a learner's developing knowledge and skills to a defined standard using both the expectations established by their program and their own expectations.

For effective learning to take place, there should be an *education alliance* between teacher and learner. This model evolved from the concept of the psychotherapeutic alliance during counselling. In the close one-to-one supervision that occurs during perinatal care shifts, teachers transmit instruction and guidance in this educational alliance. Personal interaction with the learner can be used to help demonstrate understanding and respect of their individuality, worldview, and goals—and of interpersonal boundaries. This educational alliance can help mitigate the power differentials and potentially intrinsic conflicts between the roles of teacher, role model, and assessor exposed in workplace-based evaluation (Telio et al., 2016).

WORKPLACE-BASED ASSESSMENT

The perinatal care environment lends itself well to workplace-based assessment, given that teachers and learners work side by side in antenatal clinics, labour and delivery units, and on the postpartum floor. This allows for multiple opportunities for the teacher to observe the learner and provide verbal and written feedback. Each individual interaction enhances learning—and then gets collated with the rest to provide a conclusion for the learner at the completion of their rotation with the teacher (Barrett et al., 2015).

Features of Workplace-Based Assessment

Workplace-based assessment involves sequentially observed clinical performances and encounters in a real-world setting and a well-designed system for the collection, management, and synthesis of the evaluations of these performances and encounters, which can be paper-based or online.

The process of workplace-based assessment can be encapsulated with the acronym RX-OCR:

- **R** – Establish **rapport** between learner and teacher (see education alliance above)

- **X** – Set **expectations** for the encounter, including the learner's personal goals
- **O** – **Observe** the learner's work
- **C** – Engage in a **coaching conversation**: tell learners what you observed, provide specific, actionable suggestions for improvement, and explain how these can be accomplished
- **R** – **Record** a summary of your encounter on an observation form (Gofton et al., 2017)

Some skills may be left unassessed due to the opportunistic nature of perinatal care, despite program requirements. Some of these skills may be evaluated with simulations (see Chapter 4).

Learners should be evaluated for their resilience and adaptability, not just their performance. This is appropriate because many perinatal care skills are attitudinal—related to communication skills and work ethic—not just issues of book knowledge.

Teachers will each have their own individual perspectives and priorities, leading to a range of observations for each learner. This provides for rich variety in feedback and should not be a source of concern for the individual teacher, as each evaluation is a small component of the learner's overall final report.

Because of self-reported inexperience, younger perinatal care providers may lack confidence in evaluating learners. However, no matter what, they almost certainly have more exposure to perinatal care than their learners. They are also much closer to their own experiences of learning, so they may have particularly valuable information and suggestions to impart.

FEEDBACK

Feedback is "specific, non-judgmental information comparing a learner's performance with a standard, with intent to improve performance" (Van de Ridder et al., 2008). It is the first step in the assessment process. It is primarily a verbal interaction that occurs periodically during learner-teacher interactions, in which the learner is offered suggestions to enhance knowledge, skills, or attitudes based on the teacher's experience.

Characteristics of Effective Feedback

- Based on direct observation, usually at the time of direct patient interaction (Atkinson et al., 2021)
- Timely, clear, and limited in quantity
- Focused on an aspect of performance, including communication skills, clinical reasoning, or the performance of select procedures
- Includes questions aimed at advancing clinical reasoning (Rubenstein & Talbot, 2013)
- Delivered in an empathetic manner by a trusted or respected individual (Telio et al., 2015)

Providing Feedback

Feedback is most effective when learners receive concrete, specific information about a task and how to improve their knowledge or skills. It should focus on behaviours and not be judgmental. Based on recent coaching-based models, a suggested five-step approach is . . .

1. Establish your relationship with the learner and clarify its intent as an education alliance
2. Clarify the learners' goals so that your feedback helps them attain them
3. Ask the learner about their perception of how they might improve
4. Brainstorm with learners to develop an approach to how to improve
5. Trust and coach learners to use the constructive information provided to them (Brown & Cooke, 2009)

Challenges To Effective Feedback

- It is difficult to say the right thing in the optimal fashion and convince the listener of its truth or value—especially if that information is discordant with the learner's self-image—in which case feedback can fail to modify behaviour or performance
- Feedback can be counterproductive without mutual trust, respect, and the understanding that its purpose is to help the learner

- Feedback offered bedside can be constructive, but may impact the patient's trust of the learner—offering feedback in a private setting is helpful
- Effective feedback should be considering the learner's psyche carefully in order to ensure a positive learning experience—especially when the content is difficult in one or more ways
- Expectations of the learner may be unclear from the outset
- Observations by the teacher may not match the perceptions or recollections of the learner
- Learners prefer positive feedback rather than corrective information

Example:

During an early antenatal visit for a pap smear, you observe that the medical student's examination, including speculum insertion, is uncomfortable for the patient. You then provide feedback.

Based on direct observation:

Avoid: "I heard from the nurse that the patient was uncomfortable during that pap smear."

Preferred: "Based on my observation during the pap smear, let's review that procedure together."

Well-timed:

Avoid: "Let's discuss that pap smear later."

Preferred: "Let's take a moment to review the vaginal exam now."

Non-judgmental:

Avoid: "You were insensitive to that patient's discomfort."

Preferred: "The patient seemed uncomfortable. Let's review techniques to ensure patient comfort."

Empathetic:

Avoid: "You must have felt the patient's discomfort. You couldn't miss it."

Preferred: "That was a challenging exam. I sensed you were aware of the patient's discomfort."

Using questioning:

Avoid: "Let me tell you about the pelvic anatomy—you need to know that to do a better examination."

Preferred: "Let's review this anatomy diagram together to create a method you can use that will result in less discomfort for the patient."

FORMATIVE ASSESSMENT

The next step is formative assessment—a selective subset of the feedback provided to learners during their time working with a teacher. It is documented in a formal manner by the teacher for the purpose of aggregation at the end of the learning experience or for sharing with other supervisors. Scoring of performance is often a component of formative assessment. Learners should be encouraged to initiate these formative assessments, based on their own perceived learning needs.

Example:

A family medicine resident is working with you on call for a 24-hour shift in labour and delivery. You have worked with her previously and know she is very responsible and reliable. When you first meet with her at 9 a.m., she asks you to focus the end-of shift assessment on her technical skills, as she feels still unsure of herself in suturing and artificial rupture of membranes. It ends up being a very busy shift, so there is little time for feedback. But because she asked you to complete a formative assessment at the start of the shift, you are determined to sit down with her before you leave for the office. You focus your assessment on the perineal suturing and the artificial rupture of membranes completed by her at a delivery early that morning.

It is unrealistic that all feedback provided to a learner be documented. Not only are there the barriers of time and fatigue, but too much information can lead to cognitive overload on the part of both the teacher and the learner. There are several things to consider here:

- Verbal feedback should be provided first, so that the written documentation is not a surprise to the learner.
- Due to its greater sense of permanence, written records need to be completed with attention to the learner's psyche—particularly when it comes to difficult content.
- Selected components of the feedback should be systematically documented via an online or paper-based record.
- The assessments the learner receives should be collected through a computerized system that can collate them to create a concise narrative for the end of their rotation.

Rating Scales

- **Traditional Likert scales** (Jamieson, 2004): scales in which performance is evaluated on a multipoint scale ranging from poor to excellent, usually with numerals attached to each ranking (where poor =1, excellent=5)
- **"Action-oriented" scales** (Lyons, 2009): simple scales based on expectations of graduating learners that use the following four benchmarks (see Fig. 1 for more):
  - No need for action by the teacher
  - Watchful waiting and minimal action by the teacher
  - Specific action by the teacher required
  - Intensive action by the teacher required
- **Entrustment scales** (Goften et al., 2017): In the evolving era of competency-based education, where curriculum is defined around specific clinical and professional tasks (rather than the length of training), performance is assessed by the amount of supervision required by the teacher during a period of observation, using the following anchor categories:
  - The teacher had to do it
  - The teacher had to talk the learner through it
  - The teacher had to prompt the learner from time to time
  - The teacher needed to be in the room, just in case
  - The teacher did not need to be present

Challenges With Scales. There is a tendency to focus formative feedback on what was done well or what can be constructively addressed. It is much more challenging to have the difficult conversations that document negative attitudes and behaviours. Some residents perceive that *any* documentation with negative connotations will forever be on their record, leading to them being defensive and resistant to the feedback. It could even potentially lead to them opposing the retainment of the record. It is important to remind the learner that any individual evaluation is one of *many*—and that constructive feedback is readily offset by the demonstration of progress.

A commonly used document for formative evaluation is a field note. See Figure 1 for a sample field note, specific for perinatal and newborn care. It includes antenatal, intrapartum and postpartum skills.

Perinatal and Newborn Field Note				
Antepartum	**Not applicable/ observed**	**Does not do this**	**Is starting to do this**	**Does this**
1. Provides pre-conception counselling				
2. Confirms/dates pregnancies				
3. Performs early pregnancy counselling				
4. Completes antenatal sheets				
5. Detects early pregnancy concerns				
6. Manages late pregnancy complications				
Intrapartum				
7. Diagnoses rupture of membranes				
8. Performs accurate cervical exams				
9. Manages labour, fetal surveillance				
10. Places scalp electrode correctly				
11. Performs amniotomy				
12. Manages augmentation of labour				
13. Manages a spontaneous delivery				
14. Participates in assisted vaginal delivery				
15. Performs perineal repair				
16. Communicates effectively				
Postpartum				
17. Provides lactation support				
18. Manages key issues (mother/baby)				
19. Communicates effectively				
COMMENTS:				
What was done well:				
What could be done differently:				

FIGURE 1: PERINATAL AND NEWBORN CARE FIELD NOTE.

See Figure 2 for a completed example of the above paper field note. In this example, the learner has completed several procedures (the insertion of Cervidil, the performance of cervical assessment, and assisting in a normal vaginal delivery and perineal repair). They have been provided detailed comments and a rating of their performance.

Perinatal and Newborn Field Note				
Antepartum	**Not applicable/ observed**	**Does not do this**	**Is starting to do this**	**Does this**
1. Provides pre-conception counselling	X			
2. Confirms/dates pregnancies	X			
3. Performs early pregnancy counselling	X			
4. Completes antenatal forms	X			
5. Detects early pregnancy concerns	X			
6. Manages late pregnancy complications	X			
Intrapartum				
7. Diagnoses rupture of membranes	X			
8. Performs accurate cervical exams				X
9. Manages labour, fetal surveillance			X	
10. Performs scalp electrode correctly	X			
11. Performs amniotomy	X			
12. Manages augmentation of labour			X	
13. Manages a spontaneous delivery	X			
14. Participates in assisted vaginal delivery	X			
15. Performs a perineal repair			X	
16. Communicates effectively				X
Postpartum				
17. Provides lactation support	X			
18. Manages key issues (mother, baby)	X			
19. Communicates effectively	X			

COMMENTS:

What was done well:
Complete and accurate case presentation after careful review of the antenatal records and speaking to patient. Successful and independent insertion of Cervidil for induction of labour. Followed patient closely with serial cervical exams. Attendance at delivery, assisted SVD. Started perineal repair.

What could be done differently:
We talked about discretion after a physical exam with soiled gloves to avoid upsetting patients and families.

FIGURE 2: A SAMPLE COMPLETED FIELD NOTE.

SUMMATIVE ASSESSMENT

There is a requirement for a final assessment to determine the learner's successful attainment of the expectations during any rotation. This summative assessment may be combined with a written test or may be based on workplace-based assessment alone. Summative assessment is an aggregate of the formative feedback submitted by teachers during the time the learner works in a given setting.

Each learner should have a specific teacher responsible for the overall summative assessment for the educational experience. There might be program-dependent formal or informal meetings with the teachers' group to discuss individual learners and gather impressions regarding their progress. The aggregation of the formative feedback documents serves to support these impressions and guide further decisions. Here are some of the important things to consider here:

- Teachers in a perinatal care environment should have submitted sufficient formative assessments
- The program then assembles these assessments into an aggregate report, either periodically or at the end of the educational experience, in order to provide a summary
- Each program should establish the minimum skills learners must master. These may depend on the nature of the birthing environment, the experiences available to the learners, and the institution's objectives for training.

Challenges With Summative Assessments

- Assessments risk being subjective or influenced by personality conflicts and personal biases—which interfere with fair evaluation. This can be mitigated by having an adequate number of formative assessments completed by many different teachers.
- Teachers may be hesitant to provide feedback for a learner in difficulty. Thus, there may be inadequate formative assessments to support the conclusion that the learner truly *is* in difficulty. Given negative observations about a specific learner, a teacher may feel pressured to validate

these concerns and—as a potential result—avoid documenting them at all, hoping someone else will report them.

- There is a tendency to avoid labelling a learner as having failed a rotation

See Figure 3 for a sample completed summative evaluation form. The numbers listed in each line represent the total number of field notes completed for the learner for each anchor and the corresponding ratings.

Summative Evaluation Form				
Antepartum	**Total**	**Does not do this well**	**Is starting to do this well**	**Does this well**
1. Provides pre-conception counselling	2	0	0	2
2. Confirms/dates pregnancies	3	0	1	2
3. Performs early pregnancy counselling	3	0	2	1
4. Completes antenatal form	4	0	2	2
5. Detects early pregnancy concerns	3	0	1	2
6. Manages late pregnancy complications	0	0	0	0
Intrapartum				
7. Diagnoses rupture of membranes	4	0	0	4
8. Performs accurate cervical exams	11	0	5	6
9. Manages labour, fetal surveillance	11	0	7	4
10. Places scalp electrode correctly	4	1	2	1
11. Performs amniotomy	6	0	1	5
12. Manages augmentation of labour	7	0	3	4
13. Manages a spontaneous delivery	3	1	2	0
14. Participates in assisted vaginal delivery	3	1	2	0
15. Performs perineal repair	6	0	4	2
16. Communicates effectively	10	0	0	10
Postpartum				
17. Provides lactation support	2	0	1	1
18. Manages key issues (mother/baby)	2	0	1	1
19. Communications effectively	5	0	1	4
COMMENTS:				

FIGURE 3: A SAMPLE COMPLETED SUMMATIVE EVALUATION FORM.

MULTI-SOURCE FEEDBACK (360-DEGREE EVALUATION)

As a mechanism to enhance self-assessment, multi-source feedback is the gathering of predominantly behavioural performance information from multiple peers and other collaborating professionals—and sometimes patients, too—via a confidential evaluation of an individual. This then gets organized and presented to provide insights that might be otherwise inapparent (Sargeant et al., 2007).

Multi-source feedback . . .

- Is best used for assessing interpersonal and team performance in learning environments
- Is described graphically by the term "360-degree evaluation," which gets at the way this type of feedback is gathered from those both hierarchically above and below the learner, as well as their peers
- Is typically used for a select sample of learners—usually, those who may require further insight into their evaluation
- Can provide a learner with significant insight into their personal qualities and areas in which they need development

See Figure 4 for a sample 360-degree evaluation survey

360-Degree Evaluation Survey

Instructions: Please complete the following anonymous survey to provide feedback to the learner with whom you worked. Your answers will be compiled with feedback from several other sources.

Qualities	Exceeds Expectations	Consistently meets expectations	Requires development to meet expectations
Teamwork (ability to lead and/or follow others, respect and support for co-workers)			
Adaptability (ability to manage change)			
Commitment to personal development			
Effective management of professional resources			
Dependability/reliability			
Level-headedness (i.e., keeping calm when faced with stressors)			
Follows organizational policies, and procedures			
Openness to feedback			
Effective delivery of feedback			
Responsiveness to communication			
Effective management and prioritization of responsibilities			
Commitment to professional role			

FIGURE 4: A SAMPLE 360-DEGREE EVALUATION.

TEACHER EVALUATIONS

Teacher evaluation is a key part of quality improvement in the instruction process. In a teacher evaluation, data is collected from learners regarding their experience with individual teachers. They are intended to provide constructive feedback to them (Nation et al., 2011).

The aggregated information can . . .

- Enhance teachers' awareness of their teaching styles and their impact on the learner
- Provide an avenue to inform teachers about their listening skills when it comes to their learners' ideas, thoughts, and questions

Challenges With Teacher Evaluations
- In perinatal care, there are often brief and limited interactions between learners and teachers. To maintain anonymity and provide a well-rounded perspective, a minimum number of completed learner evaluations for a given teacher is usually required (no less than five, in most cases).
- Caution is needed to interpret learners' evaluations when a personal conflict with the teacher may have negatively impacted their teacher evaluation

See Figure 5 for a sample generic teacher evaluation form.

Teacher Daily Evaluation						
	Poor	Fair	Good	Very Good	Outstanding	
Overall rating of the teacher today:						
	Strongly Disagree	Disagree	Neutral	Agree	Strongly Agree	Not Applicable
1. Allowed me to focus on my objectives						
Comments:						
2. Provided teaching appropriate to the clinical environment.						
Comments:						
3. Enabled me to enhance my procedural skills						
Comments:						
4. Supervision was appropriate for my level of training and skill.						
Comments:						
5. Challenged me and allowed me to identify areas for development.						
Comments:						
6. I was included in the team.						
Comments:						
7. Provided useful feedback.						
Comments:						
8. Was an effective role model.						
Comments:						

FIGURE 5: A SAMPLE GENERIC TEACHER EVALUATION FORM.

PROGRAM EVALUATION

Program evaluation is the collection, analysis, and reporting of factors that make a site work well for learning and those that need improvement. It is mainly intended to improve the quality of learning. Program evaluations are those that focus on the teaching and learning environment, its resources, and team functionality therein.

A well-organized and supportive learning environment can contribute to satisfying learners, attracting them to the provision of perinatal care, and fostering every participant's ability to provide safe and effective care to patients. The information gleaned from program evaluation can direct a program's priorities to support its improvement. Once the data is collated, teachers should review the content together and discuss options for change.

Challenges With Program Evaluation
- The information gathered from program evaluations is solely dependent on the subjective observations and insights of learners
- The information provided in these evaluations relates to learner satisfaction and usually does not provide any information regarding the actual learning the program fosters or the ultimate social impact it has
- Learners may not feel confident that the information they provide can lead to change
- Effective change in response to the information collected can take time to implement—and may be imperceptible to any current learners in the workplace

See Figure 6 for a sample shift evaluation form that can be completed by the learner after each day in the birthing unit.

There may also be a need to consider learners' evaluations of the overall perinatal care experience.

See Figure 7 for a sample generic rotation evaluation form.

Perinatal Care Shift Evaluation Form

1. Please rate the statements that follow with regards to your experience on this shift on a scale from "strongly disagree" to "strongly agree."	N/A	Strongly Disagree	Disagree	Agree	Strongly Agree
a) There was a specific teacher assigned and available to me for mentoring and support.					
b) I was provided with appropriate learning opportunities to reach the various competencies expected of me.					
c) There was adequate autonomy (i.e., an appropriate level of supervision) for my level of training.					
d) I received teaching appropriate to my level of training.					
e) I received useful feedback that was documented on a field note.					
f) I experienced a friendly environment where I felt I was integrated into the team.					
g) I felt that clinical and service responsibilities were apportioned appropriately between the other learners.					

h) I had a positive experience collaborating with and learning from the labour and delivery staff.					
i) I observed professional behaviour on the part of the healthcare team.					

2. The number of cases in which I participated this shift was:
3. Did a teacher observe you at least once during the shift (taking a history, discharging the patient, or any part of the physical exam?)   (Y/N)
4. Overall rating of the shift today: Poor   Fair   Good   Outstanding
5. What was your best experience today?
6. What constructive comment about the program could you offer that would have contributed to improving your experience today?
7. Was there any individual today who you would nominate for a teaching award?

FIGURE 6: A SAMPLE SHIFT EVALUATION FORM.

ROTATION EVALUATION FORM

OBJECTIVES/EXPECTATIONS/COMPETENCIES

1. Were learning objectives/expectations discussed at the onset of the rotation?
   ◯ No ◯ Yes
2. Did this rotation provide adequate opportunity for you to attain your expected competencies?
   ◯ No ◯ Yes
3. Was the teacher aware of the objectives for this rotation?
   ◯ No ◯ Yes

TEACHING, FEEDBACK, AND PERFORMANCE ASSESSMENT

	N/A	Needs major review	Needs minor reviews	Accept-able	Above average	Excellent
4. Rate the overall quality of teaching in this rotation:	◯	◯	◯	◯	◯	◯
5. Rate the acces-sibility of the staff in this rotation:	◯	◯	◯	◯	◯	◯
6. Rate the quality of the formal teaching (e.g., seminars) in this rotation:	◯	◯	◯	◯	◯	◯
7. Rate the quality of feedback you received in this rotation:	◯	◯	◯	◯	◯	◯

8. Did you have a mid-point evaluation?
   ◯ No ◯ Yes

CLINICAL/ACADEMIC ENVIRONMENT

	N/A	Needs major review	Needs minor reviews	Accept-able	Above average	Excellent
9. Rate the teaching/ service balance in this rotation:	◯	◯	◯	◯	◯	◯
10. Rate the appropri-ateness of the patient mix and volume in this rotation:	◯	◯	◯	◯	◯	◯
11. Rate the appropriateness of the level of your clinical responsibility in this rotation:	◯	◯	◯	◯	◯	◯
12. Strengths:						
13. Weaknesses:						
Additional Comments:						

FIGURE 7: A SAMPLE ROTATION EVALUATION FORM.

REFERENCES

Atkinson, A., Watling, C.J. & Brand, P.L.P. (2021). Feedback and coaching. European Journal of Pediatrics, 181, 441-446. https://doi.org/10.1007/s00431-021-04118-8

Barrett, A., Galvin, R., Steinert, Y., Scherpbier, A., O'Shaughnessy, A., Horgan, M., & Horsley, T. (2015). A BEME (Best Evidence in Medical Education) systematic review of the use of workplace-based assessment in identifying and remediating poor performance among postgraduate medical trainees. Medical Teacher, 4(1), 1-6. https://doi.org/10.1186/s13643-015-0056-9

Brown, N., & Cooke, L. (2009). Giving effective feedback to psychiatric trainees. Advances in Psychiatric Treatment, 15(2), 123-128. https://doi.org/10.1192/apt.bp.106.003293

Gofton, W., Dudek, N., Barton, G., & Bhanji, F. (2017). Workplace-Based Assessment Implementation Guide: Formative tips for medical teaching practice. 1st ed. (PDF) Ottawa: The Royal College of Physicians and Surgeons of Canada, pg. 1-12.

Jamieson, S. (2004). Likert scales: how to (ab)use them. Medical Education, 38, 1212-1218

Lyons, J.S. (2009). Communimetrics: A communication theory of measurement in human service settings. Communimetrics: A Communication Theory of Measurement in Human Service Settings, 2009, 1–224. https://doi.org/10.1007/978-0-387-92822-7

Nation, J.G., Carmichael, E., Fidler, H., & Violato, C. (2011). The development of an instrument to assess clinical teaching with linkage to CanMEDS roles: A psychometric analysis. Medical Teacher, 33(6), e290-6. https://doi.org/10.3109/0142159X.2011.565825

Rubenstein, W., & Talbot, Y. (2013). Medical Teaching in Ambulatory Care. Third Edition. University of Toronto Press, 33-38.

Sargeant, J., Mann, K., Sinclair, D., Van Der Vleuten, C.P.M., & Metsemakers, J. (2007). Challenges in multisource feedback: intended and unintended outcomes. Medical Education, 41(6), 583–591. https://doi.org/10.1111/j.1365-2923.2007.02769.x

Telio, S., Regehr, G., & Ajjawi, R. (2016). Feedback and the educational alliance: examining credibility judgements and their consequences. Medical Education, 50(9), 933–942. https://doi.org/10.1111/medu.13063

van de Ridder, J.M.M., Stokking, K.M., McGaghie, W.C., & ten Cate, O. (2008). What is feedback in clinical education? Medical Education, 42(2), 189–197. https://doi.org/10.1111/j.1365-2923.2007.02973.x

INDEX

Please note that an italicized "*f*" after a page number refers to a figure followed by its relevant number.

www.ingramcontent.com/pod-product-compliance
Lightning Source LLC
Chambersburg PA
CBHW040952170526
45159CB00013B/3105